AIDS-RELATED PSYCHOTHERAPY

(PGPS-165)

Pergamon Titles of Related Interest

Belar/Deardorff/Kelly THE PRACTICE OF CLINICAL
HEALTH PSYCHOLOGY

Dershimer COUNSELING THE BEREAVED

DiMatteo/DiNicola ACHIEVING PATIENT COMPLIANCE:
The Psychology of the Medical Practitioner's Role

Hersen/Kazdin/Bellack THE CLINICAL PSYCHOLOGY HANDBOOK

Holzman/Turk PAIN MANAGEMENT: A Handbook of
Psychological Treatment Approaches

Karoly/Jensen MULTIMETHOD ASSESSMENT OF CHRONIC PAIN

Russell STRESS MANAGEMENT FOR CHRONIC DISEASE

Watson/Greer PSYCHOSOCIAL ISSUES IN MALIGNANT DISEASE

Watson/Greer/Thomas PSYCHOSOCIAL ONCOLOGY

Winett/King/Altman HEALTH PSYCHOLOGY AND
PUBLIC HEALTH: An Integrative Approach

Related Journals
(Free sample copies available upon request)

CLINICAL PSYCHOLOGY REVIEW
INTERNATIONAL JOURNAL OF NURSING STUDIES
SOCIAL SCIENCE AND MEDICINE

AIDS-RELATED PSYCHOTHERAPY

MARK G. WINIARSKI
Montefiore Medical Center/
Albert Einstein College of Medicine

PERGAMON PRESS

Member of Maxwell Macmillan Pergamon Publishing Corporation
New York • Oxford • Beijing • Frankfurt
São Paulo • Sydney • Tokyo • Toronto

Pergamon Press Offices:

U.S.A.	Pergamon Press, Inc., Maxwell House, Fairview Park, Elmsford, New York 10523, U.S.A.
U.K.	Pergamon Press plc, Headington Hill Hall, Oxford OX3 0BW, England
PEOPLE'S REPUBLIC OF CHINA	Pergamon Press, Xizhimenwai Dajie, Beijing Exhibition Centre, Beijing, 100044, People's Republic of China
FEDERAL REPUBLIC OF GERMANY	Pergamon Press GmbH, Hammerweg 6, D-6242 Kronberg, Federal Republic of Germany
BRAZIL	Pergamon Editora Ltda, Rua Eça de Queiros, 346, CEP 04011, Paraiso, São Paulo, Brazil
AUSTRALIA	Pergamon Press Australia Pty Ltd., P.O. Box 544, Potts Point, NSW 2011, Australia
JAPAN	Pergamon Press, 8th Floor, Matsuoka Central Building, 1-7-1 Nishishinjuku, Shinjuku-ku, Tokyo 160, Japan
CANADA	Pergamon Press Canada Ltd., Suite 271, 253 College Street, Toronto, Ontario M5T 1R5, Canada

Library of Congress Cataloging in Publication Data

Winiarski, Mark G., 1950–
    AIDS-related psychotherapy / by Mark G. Winiarski.
      p.   cm. -- (Pergamon general psychology series)
    Includes bibliographical references.
    Includes index.
    ISBN 0-08-037913-3 :
    1. AIDS (Disease)--Patients--Mental health. 2. Psychotherapy.
[1. Acquired Immunodeficiency Syndrome--therapy. 2. Psychotherapy.]
I. Title. II. Series.
    [DNLM: WD 308 W772a]
RC607.A26W57 1991
616.97 '92--dc20
DNLM/DLC   90-7549
for Library of Congress   CIP

Printing: 1 2 3 4 5 6 7 8 9   Year: 1 2 3 4 5 6 7 8 9 0

Printed in the United States of America

 The paper used in this publication meets the minimum requirements of American National Standard for Information Sciences—Permanence of Paper for Printed Library Materials, ANSI Z39.48-1984

Contents

Part 4: Other HIV-Related Issues

Part 5: Resources

Preface

In 1987, when I began full-time work at St. Clare's Spellman Center for HIV-Related Disease in Manhattan, I attended numerous seminars to learn about AIDS-related psychotherapy. I had many questions: Is therapy with HIV-positive persons different from other psychotherapy? What issues arise? How can I prepare myself? I found that this work was being defined as it was being done, and that practitioners were few in number. There were not many answers; we had to follow a few guidelines and believe in our intuitions. The fear in our hearts was what had to be mastered.

Since, a small but growing number of publications and professional seminars have become available to the psychotherapist who deals with HIV-related issues. Authors are attempting to organize what we are slowly learning.

In the meantime, many psychotherapists have dared to work on this frontier, replacing fear with courage, hatred with regard, and prejudice with knowledge. While we await a medical cure, we help heal; we help a client come to terms, and to feel connected.

When I mention healing, I do not mean it in some dreamy, metaphysical sense. We do not lay on hands, at least not in any ritualistic sense, although we may touch. Therapists do not baptize, bless or otherwise assure entrance into another world or even happiness in this world. I use the word healing in the sense of restoring connection. We provide a relationship. Yalom (1980) wrote:

> It is the relationship that heals. . . . If any single fact has been established by psychotherapy research, it is that a positive relationship between patient and therapist is positively related to therapy outcome. Effective therapists respond to their patients in a genuine manner; they establish a relationship that a patient perceives as safe and accepting; they display a nonpossessive warmth and a high

degree of accurate empathy and are able to 'be with' or 'grasp the meaning' of a patient (p. 401).

This book is about both competence and healing. Many, including many would-be therapists, may believe that compassion is enough to do competent psychotherapy. In fact, compassion without competence is insufficient in any psychotherapy practice, especially in any practice with the complex issues of HIV infection. For one to say, "I have compassion, so I'll find an HIV-positive client" and to not also seek special training is unethical. One goal of this book is to provide information that would help the psychotherapist anticipate and prepare for the complexities and challenges in this special area.

AIDS-related psychotherapy serves the living, and cannot be reduced to death and dying. This is especially true as we realize that HIV-related illness is more and more a chronic condition. Although some persons with AIDS may enter psychotherapy saying they want to deal with their fear of death, more likely they will work on their fear of living with HIV infection. They will learn that life continues, albeit altered, but that when we learn how to live, then we will be more comfortable with death.

In this brief book, I introduce HIV-related psychotherapy as a subspecialty that shares commonalities with other therapies, but is also unique because of the emotional, physical, and sociopolitical aspects of HIV-related conditions. I try to provide some understanding for these issues. HIV-positive status means a future that can be improved by emotional stamina, commitment to good self-care and the seeking of competent medical care, explorations of anxiety and the past, and willingness to see life in the sharp relief it achieves when contrasted with nonlife. These years can be both terrifying and replenishing, for both client and therapist.

Let me anticipate the question, "What is the most important thing to know about this work?" The most important aspect to this work, taught me by clients, colleagues, and supervisors, was to realize that one cannot be "tough"—that one has to be vulnerable. The therapist or other health care provider cannot develop a thick skin or calloused heart. We cannot hear the news of sickness and death with a defensive shrug. That posture separates the caregiver from the client and, perhaps worse, it separates the caregiver from himself or herself. It keeps us distant from the pain, the fears, and it keeps us from being truly alive.

Whenever I write or speak publicly, I communicate the voices of the many persons with HIV infection who have shared their lives with me as psychotherapy clients, along with those who have been acutely ill and have let me sit by their beds. If there seems to be a bias toward acute illness in this writing, it is because of the impact of the bedside hospital work that I was able to do at the Spellman Center. (I am now doing outpatient-related work at Montefiore Medical Center, in the Bronx.)

Among the voices is that of one man, who died in December, 1989. Just a week before his death, I was sitting at his bedside when a nurse entered and asked what liquids he had that day. He replied, "A glass of juice, one cup of coffee, a bottle of champagne." And there also is the man who said goodbye to me with, "I'll see you when I see you." I want to thank them for teaching me about living. I wish I could name them.

I also would like to acknowledge and thank the colleagues whose lives evidence their commitment to caring for others.

My wife, Diane Sturm Winiarski, a registered nurse and home care expert, provided love, support and advice and was patient with my writing absences for almost a year. Many people reviewed the drafts and offered helpful advice. They included Gil Tunnell, PhD, of New York University Medical Center–Bellevue Hospital, and Philip R. Muskin, MD, of Columbia-Presbyterian Medical Center, my clinical supervisors; and Wallace A. Kennedy, PhD, my major professor at Florida State University, Tallahassee. Sharon Berry, PhD, of Children's Memorial Hospital, Chicago, extensively reviewed the manuscript, as did Peter A. Selwyn, MD, and Kenneth Cochrane, PhD, of Montefiore Medical Center/Albert Einstein College of Medicine.

Others who generously shared their expertise included my colleagues at the Spellman Center: Ursuline Sister Pascal Conforti, pastoral counselor; Carolyn Moorhead, RN, an analytically trained psychotherapist; Joseph Leoni, MD, neurologist; Bruce Lockhart, MD, physician; Mario Andriolo, DDS, and Roger Wills, DDS, the director of Spellman's dental clinic and his associate; Tom Watson, a resource expert, and Xena Hoffman, MS, an Albert Einstein College of Medicine/Yeshiva University graduate student in health psychology. I was also helped by Rex Swanda, PhD, neuropsychologist at New York University Medical Center-Bellevue Hospital; Deborah Orr, PhD, Westchester County Medical Center; Phillip R. Godding, PhD, Department of Veterans Affairs Medical Center, Jackson, MS; Martin Sloane, PhD, in private practice in New York; Elaine Priscantelli, CSW, Postgraduate Center for Mental Health, New York; Rose Rivera; and Carolyn Gregory.

Abbreviations

AIDS	Acquired Immune Deficiency Syndrome
ARC	AIDS-related complex
AZT	Now called zidovudine or Retrovir, an antiviral medication
CD-4 Cell	Also known as T-4 cell
CDC	(U.S.) Centers for Disease Control
CMV	Cytomegalovirus
CNS	Central nervous system
COBRA	Consolidated Omnibus Budget Reconciliation Act
DNR	Do not resuscitate
ELISA	Enzyme-linked immunosorbent assay
FDA	(U.S.) Food and Drug Administration
HIV	Human Immunodeficiency Virus (common strain is HIV-1)
HTLV-III	Human T-lymphotropic virus type III, same as HIV-1
IVDU	Intravenous drug user
KS	Kaposi's Sarcoma
LAV	French abbreviation for lymphadenopathy-associated virus (same as HIV-1)
MAI	Mycobacterium avium intracellulare
MRI	Magnetic resonance imaging
NAC	N-acetylcysteine
NIAID	(U.S.) National Institute of Allergy and Infectious Diseases
OI	Opportunistic infection
PCP	*Pneumocystis carinii* pneumonia
PCR	Polymerase chain reaction, a test for HIV

PWA   Person with AIDS
PWArc   Person with ARC
SIDA   AIDS in Spanish, Síndrome de Inmunodeficiencia Adquirida; and
           in French, Syndróme de L'immunodéficience Acquise
SSI   Supplementary Security Income
TB   Tuberculosis

PART 1

INTRODUCTION TO HIV-RELATED ISSUES

1

Introduction

This book is about a psychotherapeutic relationship that is unlike any other: A relationship that can encourage and reveal the human spirit, but always against the stark contrast of anxieties about life, the difficulties inherent in a life-threatening chronic illness, and loss.

The book is intended as a psychotherapy guide for the practitioner willing to work with a person who has the Human Immunodeficiency Virus (HIV). It is based on the belief that this practice is an important subspecialty having several requirements: Special knowledge regarding HIV, such as transmission, prevention, and its medical and psychosocial aspects; competent performance within one's training and willingness to respond with flexibility to the client's changing circumstances; and acknowledgment that this work is stressful but, with adequate psychological self-care, can also be gratifying and self-enlightening.

The art and science of this new subspecialty is evolving as it is being performed. The newness of HIV-related psychotherapeutic work is such that I do not believe practitioners could even agree on therapeutic goals (that is, if one naively believes we agree on goals in other areas of psychotherapy). One experienced therapist has said she wants her clients to leave a session feeling better than when they began. Many would take issue with that. Others, too, have stretched far beyond what they were taught. A psychoanalytically trained psychotherapist in New York began analytic work with a person with Acquired Immune Deficiency Syndrome (AIDS), and found himself at the client's residence, washing the dying man.

Nor, necessarily, would all agree on what some practitioners have found to be a necessary component of psychotherapeutic work with HIV-positive persons: flexibility to move to different points on the paradigmatic continuum,

3

depending on the client's changing circumstances. For illustration, let us characterize psychotherapists as working on this continuum: At one end, the clinician is a very supportive and engaged caretaker. Therapy sessions are dialogues and the client, and perhaps the therapist too, feels a friendship-like relationship is involved. At the other end, the therapist is committed to promotion of self-exploration; therapy is never a dialogue and the therapist is neither praiseful nor condemnatory, but always neutral. Many practitioners have found that the HIV-positive client may require both types of therapists, and many of the types in-between, but at different times during the course of the chronic illness. It may be that, early on, self-exploration is useful, especially as it helps a client approach his or her anxieties and yearnings. It may be that as the disease progresses, the therapist may make hospital visits, conduct supportive sessions by telephone, or take a greater role in case management.

Critics of this stance may say that this amounts to an eclectic psychotherapy, such that the client actually receives no psychotherapy at all. One could argue, with some justification, that if the therapist moves from insight to problem solving or case management, it may be because he or she needs to move away from the client's suffering. However, one could also argue that rigid enforcement of formality and "frames" with HIV-positive persons may also serve the therapist's need to feel separate and, hence, safe. Motivations, of course, can be many and complex and should be investigated in one's own therapy or supervision.

This book's contents reflect this appreciation for flexibility. An attempt was made to introduce useful and provocative ideas from both cognitive-behavioral and psychodynamic orientations, as well as to broadly describe HIV-related practice. Whether predominantly concerned with psychodynamics, erroneous cognitions, case management, or psychopharmacology, the practitioner should be familiar with the issues highlighted in this book, which will enable him or her to anticipate the issues of the HIV-positive client and, hence, better manage the delivery of services.

This familiarity is especially important now because skillful medical management has begun to encourage HIV-positive persons, many not otherwise inclined to take advantage of mental health services, to consider their emotional well-being. Physicians treating HIV-positive persons, noticing some psychiatric or psychological disturbance, are making more referrals to mental health practitioners. Some HIV-positive persons have found benefit in support groups and may seek individual psychotherapy. Still others seek mental health services because of severe reactions to the stress of HIV infection. Even noninfected persons express AIDS-related anxiety. Called "worried well" (see Chapter 15), these persons too may seek professional counseling.

This book is structured to help a practitioner learn the special knowledge of this subspecialty work. Part 1 describes the complexities of the medical and sociopolitical aspects of the illness. This understanding is imperative: Imagine a client's feelings if, when confiding to the therapist a new diagnosis of cytomegalovirus (CMV) retinitis, which may involve damaged eyesight, he or she receives an uncomprehending stare in return. Chapter 2 introduces this and other opportunistic illnesses as part of a brief review of the virus, its effects on the immune system, means of transmission, and the new conceptualization of HIV illness as a spectrum of conditions—ranging from HIV-positive but asymptomatic to a diagnosis of AIDS. The medical information introduced here is perishable because medical discoveries are now announced almost weekly, but will provide bases for understanding the new announcements. The psychotherapist should continue to build knowledge with readings from professional journals.

The plight of the man who was visited at his bedside by the psychoanalytically-trained therapist must also be understood in a social and political context. The man was in a special residence in New York for persons with AIDS, one of very few such residences for persons not sick enough to be hospitalized. He likely received Supplementary Security Income and, because of Medicaid's low payments to practitioners, may have had access only to public medical clinics and hospitals. To what extent does society's perceptions about AIDS and feelings about this man's lifestyle affect the availability of social and medical care? How the political, social, and economic realities of HIV-related illness affect your client and others are important components of this psychotherapeutic subspecialty. These are reviewed in Chapter 3.

Part 2 discusses the work of HIV-related psychotherapy and underlines the importance of competence, as well as consideration of different therapist roles. A competent and tender holding of the client includes a thorough assessment that illuminates the client's medical and sociopolitical situation. This assessment enables the therapist to determine what type of therapeutic contract will be needed, and if it can be provided by this therapist or if a referral will be needed. Such an assessment is outlined in Chapter 4. The therapeutic and other themes that may emerge are outlined in Chapter 5. Reflection on these will enable the therapist to anticipate and thus better respond to the client.

Other aspects of working with these clients require the therapist to have a searching eye for the physical, psychiatric, and neuropsychological complications that come with HIV infection. In many cases, early intervention by a physician can reduce the severity of these conditions; unfortunately, in many cases, the clients and their caregivers do not respond to early warning signs. Chapter 6 concerns itself with the therapist's monitoring role, and lists physical and psychiatric symptoms that require medical intervention. Psychiatric disorders and suicide are also discussed in this chapter.

Because HIV so often affects the central and peripheral nervous systems of HIV-positive persons, and because this phenomenon has attracted so much research and clinical attention, Chapter 7 discusses the neuropsychological aspects of HIV infection. For generalists, it provides basic information; for specialists, specifically psychologists who already have neuropsychological assessment training, it offers additional information regarding assessment and instruments.

Chapter 8 suggests another aspect of the psychotherapeutic role: A consultation and case management model. With AIDS becoming redefined as a chronic condition, coordinating mechanisms such as case management, which promote high levels of functioning, will receive attention. The practitioner's role as consultant and case manager is discussed in this chapter, as are goals, problems, and service providers who comprise the client's care system.

Perhaps the most important chapters in this book are those regarding the therapist's feelings, those both brought to the psychotherapy sessions and those evoked by the clients and by their situations. As the client comes to terms with loss, so too must the therapist. Practitioners must also come to terms with their grandiosities, rescue fantasies, and the helplessness inevitably felt when confronted with this illness. Chapters 9 and 10 discuss what beliefs and feelings therapists may bring to the relationship, and those that are evoked in practitioners. Chapter 11 discusses how practitioners may care for themselves: the necessity for supervision and peer support, and thoughts about that much-discussed topic, burnout.

Part 4 acknowledges other commonly discussed complexities of HIV and AIDS including HIV screening and issues of early detection (Chapter 12); prevention counseling (Chapter 13); the special issues of the intravenous drug user (Chapter 14); psychiatric issues in the "worried well" (Chapter 15); and the much-overlooked issues of spirituality (Chapter 16).

The final section, Part 5, is meant to provoke thought and facilitate the search for additional information. For those who want to consider and plan creative changes in service delivery, Chapter 17 offers some suggestions. The Appendix lists sources of information available to therapists and clients.

Why become professionally involved in HIV-related psychotherapy? There are many reasons. AIDS is at the nexus of the most important issues of our times. At the intersection that is AIDS are manifestations of our beliefs in human dignity, and issues of how societies, states, cities, and neighborhoods regard our neighbors. At the intersection that is AIDS is poverty, alternative lifestyles, questions of religious and moral judgments, ethical issues about allocations of resources. There is the challenge of learning about, supporting, and empathizing with the most basic human emotions: courage and fear, despair and doubt, shame and guilt, and acceptance of death. There are many other reasons. I hope you will share them with me.

For my part, it has been in these always complicated and emotional therapeutic relationships that I have learned the most about myself, about my willingness to be myself, and to experience what living is about. I am sitting with a man or woman who believes life is too short, and I cannot extend that life. All my gaudy pretenses are stripped away; the mahogany-framed certificates count for little. Levine (1984) wrote about a client: "In a sense, he has now become your therapist, your doorway to yourself. He is putting you in touch with all the places of fear and holding, all the need to be someone in the world, to be right, to be in control, to be good" (p. 49).

2
Medical Issues

HIV and AIDS, the constellation of ailments caused by immune deficiency, have been recognized, labelled and treated as such for less than a decade. They are still strangers to scientists and laypersons, with new, startling revelations occurring almost daily.

The 1980s saw an exponential increase in HIV information. In the 1990s new findings will continue to challenge old hypotheses and theories. Scientists now suggest that Kaposi's Sarcoma, considered AIDS-related, may be caused by an unknown sexually transmitted agent (Beral, Peterman, Berkelman & Jaffe, 1990); an eminent French scientist suggests microbes known as mycoplasmas may contribute to the virulence of AIDS in some persons (Montagnier, 1990); and others suggest that HIV may not depend on a specific receptor, CD-4, to enter cells (Levy, 1990). Each new suggestion creates a new debate; each new debate, although initially confusing to observers, can lead to new illumination. With all the medical activity, those who do AIDS-related psychotherapy must be aware that today's "knowledge" may be tomorrow's disputed, or perhaps disproven, claim.

Little is written in concrete. Even statistics, those seemingly solid descriptors, are debated and questioned. The World Health Organization has predicted that this *enfant terrible* syndrome—a constellation of ailments caused by immune deficiency—may infect 1.1 million persons globally by 1991 (Mann, 1989). By the year 2000, if no vaccine is discovered, there may be a cumulative total of more than 6 million AIDS cases worldwide (Mann, 1989). Some 700,000 new AIDS cases may be diagnosed between 1989 and 1991 alone. Yet, many believe the actual toll will be appreciably higher, and that economic, political, technological, and medical reasons contribute to undercounting around the world, including in the United States. The pediatric AIDS

8

cases of Romania, revealed only after political upheaval, is an example of how much can be hidden from view.

Even in the United States there is little agreement about the number of persons who will be diagnosed with AIDS in the 1990s. The disagreements stem from uses of different methods of statistical projection, as well as the difficulties of determining the number of persons currently HIV-infected and the time periods between infection and AIDS diagnosis. The group of articles in the March 16, 1990 issue of the *Journal of the American Medical Association* typifies the discourse. One, reporting the application of an epidemic theory, said the AIDS epidemic peaked in 1988 and projected that the number of cases will continue to decline, reaching the range of about 200,000 (Bregman & Langmuir, 1990). Another view was provided by Gail and Brookmeyer (1990) who noted that surveys indicated perhaps 1 million persons in the United States are infected and if a large percentage develop AIDS "the estimate of 200,000 cumulative cases will fall seriously short" (p. 1538). Other writers cited military data that, extrapolated, suggest a minimum of 40,000 new HIV infections in United States adults and adolescents annually (Morgan, Curran, & Berkelman, 1990).

Other predictions include that of researchers at the Hudson Institute, a think tank, who offer a scenario of up to 30,000 new HIV infections each year through 2002, when they predict there will be 14.5 million infected persons in the United States, and 1.6 million persons with AIDS (PWAs) (Johnston & Hopkins, 1989). The United States Centers for Disease Control (CDC) predicts that 390,000 to 480,000 persons will have been diagnosed with AIDS by the end of 1993, and 285,000 to 340,000 will have died from AIDS by then. HIV-positive persons totalled 1 million in the United States in September, 1990, according to the CDC.

Qualitatively, the character of HIV-related illness has changed remarkably. Originally regarded as an acutely fatal illness, AIDS in the 1990s is being seen as a chronic condition likely to be extended by improved medical management, new medications, or new applications of known substances. But increased longevity has brought new complications and problems—AIDS-related cancers among them—which patients in the 1980s did not live long enough to see (Altman, 1990).

Some now suggest that there are at least two different manifestations of AIDS, qualitatively speaking: a more virulent, problematic and nastier manifestation experienced by intravenous drug users who may be already constitutionally weakened, or who may not have access to or may not avail themselves of medical, including prophylactic, regimens; and a better-managed AIDS experienced by individuals who have good relationships with physicians and other caregivers and who make changes that enhance health and emotional well-being (T. Lazarus, personal communication, February, 1990). Data indicate that fewer drug users survive one year past their AIDS diagnosis, compared to homosexual or bisexual men without other risk factors (Harris, 1990). More data-based comparisons may be available soon.

The 1980s saw an exponential increase in HIV information. Several journals—*AIDS* and the *Journal of AIDS,* among them—have been founded and new AIDS-related data bases and information telephone lines have been established (see Appendix). Despite the outpouring of information, however, many questions remain unanswered and no cure is yet in sight.

Even at the clinical level, AIDS-related practice has changed and continues to change—and disagreements ensue. Before mid-1989, many AIDS-related advocacy groups discouraged HIV testing, saying that the asymptomatic HIV carrier had little to gain from knowing whether he was positive. (Women had more to consider, especially if pregnancy was an issue.) Advocacy groups believed that medicine had no interventions to help the asymptomatic HIV-positive person, and that the knowledge of infection could be psychologically damaging. This all changed in mid-1989 when the National Institutes of Health announced that a double-blind study found that zidovudine, formerly called AZT (azidothymidine) and also called Retrovir, helped prevent opportunistic infections in asymptomatic HIV-positive persons (National Institute of Allergy and Infectious Diseases, 1989a). That was the first indication that effective prophylaxis was possible. Advocacy groups began to encourage HIV testing for persons at risk. But proponents of prophylactic use of zidovudine (NIAID, 1990) were joined in the debate by those who had additional questions or strongly questioned its use in symptom-free individuals (Ruedy, Schechter & Montaner, 1990; Lancet, 1990).

In the psychosocial realm, the scripts of prevention counseling likewise changed over time. At first, the term "safe sex" was used, in the belief that condoms effectively prevented infection. Then evidence of the possibility of breaks and spills required the more cautious prevention term "safer sex." Other refinements were also incorporated. Some suggested the use of only latex condoms, and others, building on research that indicated the spermicide nonoxynol-9 killed HIV in the laboratory, suggested the use of condoms with that chemical (Staff, *CDC AIDS Weekly,* 1989).

If there is any single theme in the first decade of HIV, it is that knowledge and its applications are ever-changing. Competent and conscientious psychotherapeutic practice requires that the clinician have up-to-date knowledge.

One constant remains, however. The mere mention of AIDS continues to raise fears, partly due to the public's notion that AIDS is a death sentence. More realistically now, HIV-related illness means a protracted course of considerable challenge to both physical and emotional well-being.

Individuals' anxieties too are fueled by rumors, hunts for the "drugs of the month," and the allegations that not everything that can be done is being accomplished by governmental or private industry. These concerns add to the perception that the HIV infection represents, for many, a loss of control; seeking action and answers helps reestablish a sense of control.

Because HIV-related illness presents such an admixture of the physical and emotional, the psychotherapist who works with an HIV-positive client must have a broad understanding of these relationships. The clinician must not only know how the human immunodeficiency virus commandeers a CD-4 Cell but must also know the relationship between HIV infection and existential anxiety.

This chapter provides basic medical information that will help the practitioner understand and explain the mechanics of HIV infection, as well as understand the medical situation of the HIV-positive client. Also provided are tables listing the most common HIV-related conditions and available treatments. Because knowledge is constantly changing, the practitioner is urged to seek additional information.

WHAT AIDS IS

In general terms, Acquired Immune Deficiency Syndrome—a constellation of symptoms—is the manifestation of depletion of a person's immune functioning. "Acquired" means that the person was not born with the condition.

Several years ago it was believed that it was not the virus that kills, but the opportunistic infections—called opportunistic because they take advantage of the suppressed immune system. Now, HIV-related illnesses include the direct effects of the virus as well as the effects of opportunistic infections.

Despite lack of knowledge about many specifics, the consensus is that AIDS is caused by a virus called the Human Immunodeficiency Virus (HIV), the current generally accepted name. Several types have been discovered, but the most common is HIV-1.

Earlier articles and research used other names for the virus. United States scientists, primarily Dr. Robert C. Gallo of the National Cancer Institute, had called their discovery human T-lymphotropic virus type III (HTLV-III), believing it was related to a leukemia-causing virus. In France, Luc Montagnier and colleagues of the Pasteur Institute had called their version of the virus lymphadenopathy-associated virus (LAV). In 1987, the French and U.S. governments signed an agreement giving each credit as codiscoverers of the AIDS virus (see Shilts, 1988, for an account of the rivalries between the two groups of scientists; also Crewdson, 1989, for his award-winning account that raises questions about the official scientific history of the discovery of HIV, and Crewdson, 1990, for a followup report).

The term AIDS was coined in 1982 to replace GRID, Gay-related Immune Deficiency, the earliest appellation for the constellation of symptoms. In French and Spanish-speaking parts of the world, the syndrome is called SIDA, for Síndrome de Inmunodeficiencia Adquirida in Spanish and Syndróme de L'immunodéficience Acquise in French.

HIV has likely been in North America since the 1970s. One hypothesis is that it is related to a version of an immune deficiency-causing virus found in monkeys, and that in the past 30 to 40 years a simian immunodeficiency virus may have infected a person in West Africa and evolved as an HIV strain (Hirsch, Olmsted, Murphey-Corb, Purcell, & Johnson, 1989). Some suggest that HIV was carried to African cities, and from there to other parts of the world. Others, however, note that serological studies have not proven this. "The most plausible theory is that HIV arose in Africa, perhaps mutating from a less pathogenic human virus, or crossing over from an animal population, before becoming a human pathogen," wrote Osmond (1990, p. 1.1.4-2). See also Essex and Kanki (1988) for a description of their attempts to find the origin of the AIDS virus.

IMMUNOLOGY

To understand how HIV creates immune deficiency, a brief review of the immune system, limited here to AIDS-related aspects, may be helpful.

Our immune system is our protector against "foreign invaders:" bacteria, viruses, and parasites. Now immunologists also believe the immune system protects us from mutant cells that continue to proliferate, becoming neoplasms or tumors.

The immune system, simplistically speaking, has two major branches. The first produces B-cells, which are born in the bone marrow and produce what is called humoral immunity.

The second branch, more specifically related to AIDS, is termed cell-mediated immunity and creates T-cells born in lymph nodes. There are five types of T-cells which, confusingly, have many interchangeable names. These seem to be specialized; some natural killer T-cells go after infections, others after tumors. HIV-positive persons have normal numbers of killer cells, but their ability to destroy tumor cells has been found to be impaired (Rook et al., 1985).

With AIDS, we are especially concerned about two other types of T-cells: one is the T-helper cell or T-4 cell, now also called CD-4 for the specific surface molecule which acts as a "dock" for HIV; the other is the T-suppressor cell, which "cools down" the immune response when the threat seems over. The T-cells, as well as the B-cells, are referred to as lymphocytes, the generic term for one of the basic cells of the immune system.

Also in this complicated picture are monocytes which, when they leave the blood stream and enter tissues, become macrophages. They have many functions, some not yet clearly understood. They help the body to determine what is foreign and to present antigens to lymphocytes. They also function as "Pac-man" cells that process and chew up foreign matter. They produce antimicrobial substances and antiviral interferon. (The interferon that is much in the news today as an anticancer and AIDS substance is an adjunct to our natural interferon.)

Macrophages and circulating CD-4 cells are among the first victims of the virus although specific cells of the "gastrointestinal tract, uterine cervical cells, and glial cells of the central nervous system (CNS) may also be targets" (Volberding & Cohen, 1990, p. 4.1.1-1). During the early stage of infection, a person may suffer symptoms—such as fever, swollen glands, and malaise and, in about 50% of individuals, a rash—called acute retroviral syndrome (see Crowe & McGrath, 1990, for additional information). Meanwhile the infected person's body is mounting its immune response. This response eventually produces antibodies, which are detected by the commonly used HIV tests.

VIROLOGY

HIV belongs to a group called retroviruses, and is related to a subgroup of these, called lentiviruses. Retroviruses were initially regarded as transmitters of malignant diseases, although now some have been found which do not. Lentiviruses are associated with chronic diseases.

Retroviruses are not living, but are bits of genetic material. Their composition includes two strands of single-stranded ribonucleic acid (RNA) surrounded by an envelope that helps them gain entry to different cells. HIV's envelope and surface protein help it enter other cells.

Although HIV is now believed to attack many kinds of cells by means of unknown receptors or "docks" (Levy, 1990), the infection of CD-4 cells has received the most attention. Also, the CD-4 infection and destruction of those cells has been most salient to individuals because a person's CD-4 counts, as measured by blood tests, are generally accepted markers for general immune functioning. Normal CD-4 levels are above 500 in a cubic millimeter of blood. Persons with severe HIV infection may have as few as 50, 10, or no CD-4 cells upon testing. How does this occur?

The takeover of CD-4 cells occurs gradually. The virus docks and fuses onto the cell, using a receptor site that is a perfect fit. Once fused, the viral RNA employs an enzyme called reverse transcriptase to produce, from the RNA, first a single strand and then a double strand of deoxyribonucleic acid (DNA). This DNA is called provirus and goes directly to the CD-4 cell's nucleus where it is integrated into the cell's genetic code. Only when there is a threat of a pathogen does the incorporated provirus do its work. It then transcribes new viral RNA while the infected cell divides. The messenger RNA then starts to create new viral protein and the CD-4 cell is destroyed.

Recent indications are that neither the presence of the specialized receptor site nor HIV's entry into cells is sufficient for destruction of the CD-4 cells. It may be that a pathogen, which provokes the CD-4–cell response, is a crucial but unknowing coconspirator. The CD-4 divides in response to the pathogen and is destroyed for its efforts. The net effect, then, is a decreased CD-4 count in an infected person's blood.

More recently, scientists have begun to discuss a variety of new concepts regarding HIV infection. "Initially, the T helper lymphocyte was considered the target cell for the AIDS virus and the CD-4 molecule was identified as the attachment site or receptor" for HIV, noted Levy (1990) in a presentation at the Sixth International Conference on AIDS. He added, however, that research now strongly suggests any human cell may be infected by HIV. The HIV virus may infect some cells by binding to antibodies that cannot neutralize it, he said (1990).

Moreover, Levy announced that the virus in an individual may become more virulent over time. ". . . An HIV obtained from an individual with a relatively non-symptomatic infection was different from the virus strain recovered from the same individual after development of AIDS," Levy (1990) said. "Not only do more virulent strains appear to evolve in the host over time, but viruses with distinct features can emerge in an individual after several years and show a predilection for certain tissues." Levy and his colleagues suggest a small change in the virus's genetic structure over time may be responsible.

At the same conference Montagnier (1990), the French scientist who discovered LAV, suggested that microbes known as mycoplasma may make HIV more potent. He said he has isolated the organism from the blood of a significant number of PWAs, and is now studying whether it is just an opportunistic agent or one with a more important role.

Implications of Viral Evolvement

While Levy's announcement that the virus appears to change within an individual was news, HIV's ability to change into different strains over time has caused great concern for years (Shaw et al., 1984). Additional strains, dubbed HIV-2 and HIV-3, have been found (Wong-Staal et al., 1987). The primary difference seems to be in a protein in the viral envelope (Hahn et al., 1985; Ratner, Gallo, & Wong-Staal, 1985). Because these envelopes are the most vulnerable target of antibodies, Hall (1988) noted that this may be a strategy evolved to evade destruction by a host's immune system. This change in the viral envelope also complicates the hunt for a vaccine because a vaccine that may interfere with the envelope of one strain may not destroy that of another.

TRANSMISSION

No evidence exists for HIV transmission by insect bites or by casual contact that does not involve exchange of bodily fluids. How does someone get infected by HIV? Someone contracts HIV by receiving into one's body the HIV-infected fluids of another person. (See Friedland & Klein, 1987, for an overview of transmission.)

These fluids and the usual means of transmission are:

1. Semen and vaginal and cervical secretions, shared during sex.

This occurs when fluids with virus are introduced into the body of a sex partner. Some believe the most dangerous route appears to be anal sex, because the friction causes tissue breakage, allowing greater access to the receptive partner's blood stream.

Heterosexual transmission is the predominant epidemiological pattern in central Africa and the Caribbean, while homosexual transmission and infection via intravenous drug use has been the predominant pattern in North America and Western Europe (Zuger & Steigbigel, 1990). In Africa, compared to North America, there is a larger group of infected heterosexual persons with a large number of sexual contacts. Moreover, transmission there was abetted by a relatively high incidence of genital ulcer disease, a "cofactor" believed to help HIV transmission. In North America, the initially infected group or "pool" with a large number of contacts was gay men. With decreased seroconversion rates in gay communities due to education programs, the sexual transmission focus is turning to heterosexuals. Transmission among this group in the United States "has increased both absolutely and proportionately over the last several years" (Zuger & Steigbigel, 1990, p. 3).

Some clients ask about their chances of infection over repeated instances of unprotected sexual intercourse. While statistically based risk predictions have been published for heterosexual transmission (e.g., Hearst & Hulley, 1988), others have found "a tremendous heterogeneity in infectivity: some couples experience transmission after only a few contacts, whereas other women remain uninfected despite thousands of repeated unprotected contacts" (Padian & Francis, 1988, p. 1879). Factors that may influence the chances of transmission during sexual encounters include the stage of the infected partner's illness (a person in the later stages of illness may be more infectious), the susceptibility of the currently negative partner, and conditions called "cofactors" still being studied.

Also a concern is the possibility of female-to-male or female-to-female sexual transmission of HIV. Scientists have found HIV in infected women's vaginal and cervical secretions (Wofsy et al., 1986; Vogt et al., 1987). Several cases of heterosexual transmission of HIV from woman to man have been reported in the United States (Redfield et al., 1985) but that route is still considered an exception here (Zuger & Steigbigel, 1990). Cases have been reported of female-to-female transmission with oral, anal and digital contact and exposure to vaginal blood (Marmor et al., 1986) and female-to-male via fellatio and cunnilingus (Spitzer & Weiner, 1989).

2. Blood, contained in needles or other paraphernalia shared by intravenous drug users, or transfusion with contaminated blood.

After an intravenous drug user injects a drug, blood may be left in the syringe. When this needle is shared, the second user's injection will contain a portion of the first user's blood along with the drug. If the first user's blood contains HIV, then the second person receives the HIV also. Some now believe the HIV may also be transmitted when injectors share contaminated filters or water used to wash injection equipment.

A person can also receive the virus by being transfused with contaminated blood. Before 1985 blood was not tested for HIV and a majority of those who chronically received transfusions and blood products were at great risk for infection. An official of the Hemophilia Foundation estimates that 70% of those with hemophilia are now HIV-positive.

Since about mid-1985, donated blood has been routinely screened for HIV, significantly reducing the risk of obtaining contaminated blood. Contaminated blood can evade the screening only when the donation is made after infection but before antibodies appear. With this in mind, researchers (Cumming, Wallace, Schorr, & Dodd, 1989) estimated that about 131 contaminated blood units were transfused in 1987, and a patient had odds of 1 in 153,000, per unit transfused, of contracting HIV. A patient who received the average transfusion of 5.4 units has 1 chance in 28,000 of being infected with HIV, the researchers estimated. Goedert et al. (1989) wrote, "The nearly complete elimination of new HIV-1 seroconversions since 1986 among persons with hemophilia demonstrates the effectiveness of these measures" (p. 1145).

Experts suggest that a person contemplating elective surgery discuss with the physician the possibility of storing one's own blood in the weeks before the procedure, in the event that transfusion may be needed. Receiving one's own blood is called autologous transfusion. These experts discourage "directed donations," in which family members provide blood, because of the possibility of undisclosed risk factors in those relatives.

3. In utero transmission, from an HIV-positive mother to the fetus.

The mother's fluids shared with the fetus may include HIV, the mother's antibodies, or a combination of the virus and antibodies. After birth, the newborn may test HIV-positive, but the antibodies detected may be the mother's because they cross the placenta; therefore a positive HIV test does not necessarily mean HIV infection. Scientists believe 30% to 50% of the newborns actually have the virus. The remaining children who test positive will shed their mother's antibodies within 15 months.

Occasionally a clinician encounters someone who denies any risk factors for HIV transmission. This is a stance seemingly more prevalent in middle- and upper-income communities, that sometimes abates as the client becomes more comfortable with the counselor. Ruben et al. (1989) found that 27% of HIV-infected men in Queens, New York, denied risk factors, compared to a denial rate of 6% in New York City as a whole. They found also a higher percentage of women infected through heterosexual intercourse in a Queens sample, compared to a citywide sample. They suggested that the men's denial of risk may contribute to the higher rate of heterosexual transmission.

COURSE OF INFECTION

After a person receives the virus into his or her body there is a course of infection with several substages. These substages are often described in piece-meal fashion and cause considerable confusion. Newer commentaries describe early, middle, and crisis phases of HIV-related illness (Baltimore & Feinberg, 1989).

To simplify matters, I will illustrate the stages with the case of Kathy, a woman who was infected on a Saturday night by having unprotected sex with a carrier of the AIDS virus. First, she travels through the "window of non-detectability" to a positive HIV test. Then, after an undetermined period of time of being asymptomatic—called the incubation period—she may have symptoms of HIV infection.

Window of Nondetectability

If Kathy were to be tested on the Monday after infection via unprotected intercourse with an HIV-positive partner, her test is unlikely to show infection. Some people refer to the commonly used enzyme-linked immunosorbent assay (ELISA) and Western Blot tests as the "AIDS tests," but they have nothing to do with the symptoms of AIDS, nor do they detect HIV directly.

Rather, the commonly used test is a two-step process that detects the presence of antibodies to HIV. Blood is usually drawn from the arm of the patient and is first tested with ELISA. The test detects antibodies to a number of viral proteins. If there is a positive response, signs that the antibody is present—or if there is a suspected false-negative (a negative result even if the person is infected)—the blood sample should undergo a second ELISA (Wilber, 1990). The Western Blot test is then used for confirmation. The two tests are extremely accurate. With use of ELISA and Western Blot, the rate of false-positives—signs of HIV antibody when none is present—was found to be 1 in 135,000 in a low-risk population (Burke et al., 1988). Another study found a false-positive rate of 0.0006 (MacDonald et al., 1989). When the antibody is present in peripheral (such as from the arm) blood, "the sensitivity of current-generation ELISA is close to 100 percent" (Wilber, 1990, p. 2.1. 2.-3), making false-negatives—a negative result even when the person has antibodies—extremely rare. Of course, early in the infection no antibodies may be present.

In Kathy's case, if her body has not yet produced antibodies, she will have a negative test, with the erroneous implication that she does not have the virus. With antibody testing, a window of nondetectability occurs which lasts as long as it takes for a person to develop the antibodies—believed to be as long as 6 months. If it takes Kathy 6 months to develop antibodies, she will not have a positive HIV test until then. She has a 6-month window of nondetectability;

usually, however, the window is less than 3 to 4 months. If she donates blood during that "window" period, the blood—which has the virus but not the antibodies—will test negative and be used by a blood bank.

New technology currently available can now detect the virus itself. The polymerase chain reaction test (PCR) amplifies and detects proviral DNA sequences. This test avoids the window of nondetectability but because of a tendency toward false-negatives it is still considered experimental (Cohen, 1990).

Incubation Period From Infection to Symptoms

Once Kathy is tested and antibodies are found, she is said to have "seroconverted." With seroconversion, she is "HIV-positive" or "HIV-antibody–positive." Now she is likely to go through an "incubation period" in which she has no physical symptoms. She is now "HIV-positive but asymptomatic." If she begins to have HIV-related symptoms, her asymptomatic status will change.

Scientists' knowledge about the incubation period, the time from infection to symptoms, has increased significantly since the discovery of the syndrome. This period has also lengthened because we have more history with the virus. Research data now indicate that cumulatively about 39% of gay men in San Francisco are diagnosed with AIDS by 8 years after HIV infection (Bacchetti & Moss, 1989; Lifson et al., 1989).

A study of persons with hemophilia and related disorders infected by contaminated blood products found the age at time of seroconversion to be significantly related to development of AIDS. Using actuarial methods, Goedert et al. (1989) determined that AIDS develops within 8 years of infection for 43.7% of those infected after age 34, 26.8% of those infected between ages 18 and 34, and 13.3% of those infected between ages 1 and 17. These numbers are likely to change as our experience lengthens.

AIDS DIAGNOSTIC CRITERIA

With Kathy's presentation of symptoms, her physician tries to classify her using stringent diagnostic criteria provided by the Centers for Disease Control (1987). If she meets certain criteria, she will be diagnosed with AIDS. If she falls short of that criteria, she may be told that she has HIV-related symptomatic illness. In past years, if her symptoms were HIV-related but fell short of AIDS, she may have been told she has AIDS-related complex (ARC). However, because no agreed-upon case definition of ARC was established, that term came to encompass different meanings for different physicians. "It was a soft mix of a whole batch of things" (G. Friedland, personal communication, June 29, 1990; see also Abrams, 1990).

While "ARC" may be easier to say than "HIV-related symptomatic illness," it is nevertheless now considered "no longer useful, either from a clinical or a public health perspective" (Institute of Medicine/National Academy of Sciences, 1988, p. 37) and its use is fading.

For Kathy's physician the diagnosis classification process begins with availability of laboratory evidence of HIV infection. If HIV testing was not done or was inconclusive, definitive diagnosis of any of 12 "indicator diseases" would lead to a diagnosis of AIDS if other causes for immune deficiency were absent. The indicator diseases include neoplasms, such as Kaposi's Sarcoma (KS); specific fungal or protozoan infections, or *pneumocystis carinii* pneumonia (PCP). With laboratory evidence of HIV infection, 1 of these 12 indicator diseases is cause for an AIDS diagnosis regardless of the possibility of other causes of immune deficiency. Moreover, with evidence of HIV infection, any of several other conditions would lead to an AIDS diagnosis. These include dementia, wasting syndrome, tuberculosis other than in the lungs, and recurrent salmonella in the blood.

AIDS AS A SPECTRUM OF ILLNESS

The CDC created the diagnostic criteria to increase the reliability of diagnosis and therefore to assist reporting and research efforts. While useful for epidemiologists and researchers, the conceptualization of HIV-related disease as falling neatly into one of several categories is believed by many to ignore the realities of the condition. Those realities include several clinical issues.

First, rarely is there any orderly progression of symptoms. That everyone who gets AIDS is HIV-positive is, perhaps, the only common denominator of HIV-related conditions. For some the first indication of illness may be persistent generalized lymphadenopathy, and others may have other symptoms, such as thrush, that indicate immune suppression. Yet others may have no early symptoms and learn of HIV infection only after hospitalization for a major opportunistic infection.

Second, some persons with HIV-related symptomatic illness may be sicker through a panoply of conditions—none a criterion for AIDS—than a person who has AIDS and is not suffering any current opportunistic infection (OI). In fact, with prophylactic medication for such conditions as PCP, the already-diagnosed PWA may actually be healthier than a person with a persistent symptomatic illness that is more difficult to protect against or treat.

Third, the CDC classification focuses primarily on discrete symptoms in contrast to a holistic overall picture of the patient, which should also include the emotional and psychiatric aspects.

A clinically oriented conceptualization of HIV illness includes not just strict diagnostic criteria, but rather encompasses a wide spectrum that ranges from HIV infection at one end to severe immune system compromise at the other (see Volberding & Cohen, 1990, for an extended description). In between are many shades of conditions and illnesses, which may appear singly or in combinations in any person. Within this conceptualization, scientists and clinicians can view many physical and emotional phenomena—CD-4 counts and emotional responses among them—together with the physical manifestations that comprise CDC criteria.

Besides the CDC criteria, several other systems are available to describe the health status of the HIV-positive person and, potentially, to aid in predictive efforts. Redfield, Wright, and Tramont (1986) have created the Walter Reed Staging System, which has five stages before, and one stage after, opportunistic infection. Turner, Kelly, and Ball (1989) provide a four-level staging system which hopes to predict longevity. And Yale researchers (Justice, Feinstein, & Wells, 1989) have proposed a three-stage system for AIDS patients based on physiologic deficits rather than diagnostic features.

RELATED CONDITIONS
AND OPPORTUNISTIC INFECTIONS

Persons with immune suppression caused by HIV infection are susceptible to a wide range of conditions and illnesses. Most of these are called opportunistic infections. These generally are caused by organisms found commonly in the environment but which will not cause illnesses in people with normal immune functioning. For example, persons with immune deficiency are warned to avoid contact with a cat's litter-box contents because cat feces may contain an organism that invades the nervous system, causing toxoplasmosis. Others (with the exception of pregnant women, because toxoplasmosis may injure the fetus) need not avoid cleaning the cat's litter box.

Another HIV-related phenomenon is exacerbation of illness, compared to what may occur in a noninfected individual. For example, a noninfected person may contract salmonella poisoning, which remains restricted to the gastrointestinal tract. An HIV-positive person is more likely to have salmonella spread to the blood stream, with reccurences after the first bout. Other conditions, particularly involving the nervous system, may be the direct result of HIV. HIV-infected cells can be found in the brain, lymph nodes, bone marrow, lung, skin, and bowels.

In Table 2.1 HIV-related conditions are grouped according to physical manifestations. Also listed are the causative organisms, symptoms, and treatments.

PROPHYLACTIC MEDICATIONS

When AIDS first manifested itself, whether named or not, the first battle with PCP was likely the last. The condition often was not recognized, and fewer treatments were available. Prophylactic treatments were unknown.

Many changes have occurred since. The application of effective anti-OI drugs has allowed many patients to survive one, two, even three or more bouts of PCP. Prophylactic uses of medications are being increasingly studied and have had several effects: They have delayed or prevented the target conditions, including PCP; PCP is less often the first major opportunistic infection experienced by the HIV-positive individual; and prophylactic medications apparently extend life. People infected with HIV are living longer now (Harris, 1990; Lemp, Payne, Neal, Temelso, & Rutherford, 1990) and prophylactic medications, including zidovudine, Pentamidine, Dapsone, and regimens for tuberculosis may be one reason. Zidovudine, widely used prophylactically, has perhaps attracted the most research attention. Several protocols from the U.S. National Institute of Allergy and Infectious Diseases (NIAID) (1989a) produced findings that zidovudine delayed development of symptoms in certain subgroups of asymptomatic HIV-positive persons. These reports led to the U.S. Food and Drug Administration's (FDA) approval in 1990 of use of the drug by asymptomatic persons whose CD-4-cell counts were as high as 500. Even with that approval, controversy regarding its use continued. "Scientists are not unanimous in endorsing zidovudine . . . therapy for patients . . . whose CD-4 cell counts are above 200" reported Cotton (1990, p. 1605). Questions of longterm benefit, toxicity, and resistance remain, Cotton observed. " 'Reasonable persons with the data in hand can disagree' on the value of early treatment because of all the unanswered questions" (Cotton, 1990, p. 1605; see also *Lancet,* 1990; Chapter 12).

RESEARCH TRENDS

Rules based on scientific principles and approved by the Food and Drug Administration are used in the study of drugs before they are approved for widespread use. The federally approved multistep clinical trials include these levels (NIAID, 1989b):

- In vitro (test tube) and animal studies.
- Phase One: Done with a small number of human subjects, to determine if the drug is safe.
- Phase Two: At this and the next level, volunteers are randomly assigned to treatment and control (placebo) groups. Neither the subject nor those who directly treat the patient know which group the subject is in, although someone keeps a "key," telling the group assignment. This phase tests the drug's effectiveness and short-term safety.
- Phase Three: Randomized, double-blind studies generally over 1 to 4 years to test safety, effectiveness, and dosage level.

Several safeguards are built into these procedures. Impartial committees oversee these trials to protect the interests of patients. Those who oversee the studies may end the studies early if results or problems are evident.

Table 2.1 Common HIV-Related Conditions

DERMATOLOGICAL CONDITION	ORGANISM	SYMPTOMS	TREATMENT	NOTABLE SIDE EFFECTS
Sebhhoreic dermatitis.	Unknown—may be skin fungus or yeast-related.	Rash, dandruff.	Clotrimazole or ketoconozole followed by 1% hydrocortisone.	Peeling.
GASTROINTESTINAL CONDITION	**ORGANISM**	**SYMPTOMS**	**TREATMENT**	**NOTABLE SIDE EFFECTS**
Cryptosporidiosis.	Protozoa.	Severe diarrhea.	Spiramycin under study. Diarrhea treated with loperamide, diphenoxylate with atropine, Imodium, Lomotil, Somatostatin.	None.
NEOPLASTIC CONDITIONS	**ORGANISM**	**SYMPTOMS**	**TREATMENT**	**NOTABLE SIDE EFFECTS**
Kaposi's Sarcoma (KS).	Neoplasm—may be caused by unknown sexually transmitted organism.	On skin, purplish thickening lesion; also can affect internal organs, mouth.	Chemotherapy. Immunotherapy with interferon. Radiation, cryosurgery, cosmetology.	Flu-like symptoms.
Lymphoma.	Neoplasm.	Tumor, internal.	Chemotherapy, radiation.	

Table 2.1 (Continued)

ORAL CONDITIONS	ORGANISM	SYMPTOMS	TREATMENT	NOTABLE SIDE EFFECTS
Candidiasis (oral thrush).	Fungus.	White coating in mouth which can be removed by scraping.	Clotrimazole (Mycelex) or nystatin. Ketoconazole (Nizoral) for more severe cases.	Nausea, abnormal liver function tests. Liver problems with long-term use.
Hairy leukoplakia.	Believed caused by Epstein–Barr virus.	White coating not scrapable.	Acyclovir may be used but condition is generally not treated.	Blood chemistry changes.
Herpes Simplex.	Herpesvirus.	Clear blisters that later ulcerate and coalesce.	Acyclovir.	
Major apthous ulcer.	Unknown.	Ulceration.	Topical steroids; tetracycline oral suspension.	
HIV Gingivitis.	Various bacteria.	Distinctive redness of gingiva.	Debridement, scraping; Chlorhexidine gluconate (Peridex).	
HIV Periodontis.	Various bacteria.	Soft tissue necrosis and rapid destruction of periodontal attachment and bone.	Antibiotic therapy; surgery may be indicated when conservative treatment is unsuccessful.	

NERVOUS SYSTEM CONDITIONS	ORGANISM	SYMPTOMS	TREATMENT	NOTABLE SIDE EFFECTS
Cryptococcal meningitis (crypto).	Fungus.	Headache, mutism, fever, nausea, vomiting, photophobia, mental status changes.	Fluconazole.	Headache, abdominal discomfort, elevated liver enzymes.
			Amphotericin-B.	Fever, chills; renal, liver, bone marrow effects.
Progressive multifocal leukoencephalopathy.	J.C. Papova(virus).	Focal neurological deficits, depending on lesion sites; mental status deterioration.	None.	

Table 2.1 (Continued)

	ORGANISM	SYMPTOMS	TREATMENT	NOTABLE SIDE EFFECTS
NERVOUS SYSTEM CONDITIONS				
Toxoplasmosis.	Protozoa.	Focal neurological deficits, depending on site. Fever, headache, seizures.	Pyrimethamine alone and with sulfadiazine or Leucovorin. Clindamycin.	Rash; depression of cells created in bone marrow.
RESPIRATORY CONDITIONS				
Pneumocystis carinii pneumonia.	Parasite.	Fever, cough, trouble breathing, inadequate oxygen.	Bactrim (trimethoprim-sulfamethoxazole TMP-SMX).	Rash; liver problems; nausea and vomiting. Anemia, lowered white blood count, other blood chemistry changes.
			Pentamidine. Dapsone with trimethoprim.	Renal failure, pancreatitis, diabetes, anemia, rise in creatinine, neutropenia, hyponatremia.
DISSEMINATED CONDITIONS				
Cytomegalovirus (CMV).	Herpesvirus.	In eye, affects vision and can lead to blindness. GI tract: esophagitis, gastritis, ileitis. CNS: encephalitis. Lungs: pneumonitis.	Ganciclovir (DHPG). Foscarnet. Not treatable in GI, CNS.	Neutropenia, leukopenia.

Table 2.1 *(Continued)*

DISSEMINATED CONDITIONS	ORGANISM	SYMPTOMS	TREATMENT	NOTABLE SIDE EFFECTS
Herpes simplex.	Herpesvirus.	Vesicles, ulcers, fever—prolonged illness with delayed healing. Mouth, genital, rectal areas. Esophagitis. In brain, slow or acute encephalitis with fever, headache, lethargy, confusion.	Acyclovir, Foscarnet.	Blood chemistry changes.
Herpes Zoster (Varicella-Zoster).	Herpesvirus.	Pain, localized rash, vesicles. May disseminate to lung, liver, CNS.	Acyclovir.	
Mycobacterium avium intracellulare (MAI).	Bacteria.	Malaise, fevers, night sweats, weight loss, diarrhea. May disseminate to lungs, bone marrow, blood, liver, other organs.	Rifabutin under study; clofazimine, aminoglycosides, ethambutol, ciprofloxacin. Combined regimens, none with proven efficacy.	Nephrotoxicity, optic neuritis.
Tuberculosis.	Mycobacteria.	Coughing and respiratory problems when in lungs. Pain, fever, when disseminated.	Isoniazid, rifampin. Pyrazinamide, Ethambutol.	Liver problems, neuropathy, lethargy. CNS abnormalities. Fatigue.

(Oral information: M. Andriolo, R. Wills, personal communication, December 1989. TB and MAI information from Pitta, 1990).

25

One trend in AIDS medication research is drug research occurring outside this framework. A small but increasing number of doctors (generally in New York and San Francisco) are reportedly treating patients in "private studies" which are not FDA-approved multistep clinical trials. One such trial, of Compound Q, was done secretly and became public only after several subjects died. Project Inform in San Francisco led the study, and spokespersons there, and other AIDS-patient advocates, defended the action as necessary to possibly save lives while circumventing a lengthy federal process. Critics said the private trials are unethical, in that there were inadequate safeguards for patients' rights and safety. Project Inform spokespersons indicated this trial's level of informed consent was unprecedented (Staff, November, 1989). In New York, the picture became increasingly cloudier after a newspaper reported a subject died after hospital emergency room personnel were not informed of the subject's use of the substance. Project Inform called the report "spectacularly inaccurate" (Staff, November 1989, p. 3). By March 1990 the FDA announced that the Compound Q trial could continue, but with protocol revisions (Kolata, 1990).

Another trend is a newly approved "parallel track" that enables physicians to provide medications that are the subject of research protocols to those not enrolled in those projects. Initial guidelines for participation include: The parallel track patient cannot tolerate or has failed standard therapies; no standard therapy exists for the patient's condition; the patient is too sick to travel or lives too far from a protocol site; and the patient must continue concomitant medications that may exclude him or her from clinical trials.

A third trend is the investigational use of combination regimens that employ two or three drugs concurrently. Many researchers now indicate that the future of HIV therapy lies in combination of multiple agents, which would make the best use of the favorable aspects of each and reduce unfavorable side effects.

A weekly newsletter annually publishes a directory of antiviral and immune-system–modulating treatments being used or studied (see DeNoon, 1989).

DRUG-OF-THE-MONTH PHENOMENON

Unfortunately, a phenomenon known as the drug of the month occurs regularly in communities with large numbers of HIV-infected persons. Rumors, leaks of early protocol successes, or preliminary scientific reports issued at specialty meetings promote large-scale efforts to obtain these substances. In September 1989, for example, a report from a meeting in Geneva, Switzerland, installed N-acetylcysteine (NAC) as the drug of the month. Stanford University researchers had reported testing the substance, normally used to treat bronchitis, on HIV-infected cells in a test tube.

CHRONICITY VERSUS QUALITY OF LIFE

The successes with prophylaxis as well as improved treatments of OIs and other AIDS-related conditions are extending the lives of HIV-positive persons. This raises the issue of quality of life.

James, a 50-year-old gay PWA who lives in a Polish-American enclave in New York, was prescribed several medications for his mycobacterium avium intracellulare (MAI). He complained to his therapist that he felt very lethargic, was sleeping more hours than he was awake, and became weak during short walks. During a hospitalization, when the drugs were discontinued, he recovered his energy and strength. Upon discharge, when he restarted the regimen, he again felt lethargic and weak. In psychotherapy he said he was considering discontinuing the medication. His argument: "But, you know, I'd prefer feeling better for a short while than feeling like I do now for a longer while." Others express similar concerns regarding HIV dementia and other nervous system manifestations. They are concerned that if they live longer, they may become demented or otherwise debilitated, and live longer with those conditions. Moreover, those who discuss the economies of medical treatment may argue that certain prophylactics and treatments maintain life at a very high cost, with too little return in life quality.

Sometimes clients are reluctant to discuss these concerns with their physicians, and either covertly or overtly take smaller doses or discontinue medications. When medical providers do not understand the patient's rationale and emotional concerns, they may view the person as uncooperative and noncompliant, or as wishing to die. Part of the task of psychotherapy is to enable the client to attain an informed choice, ideally after discussions with medical caregivers about length and quality of life, and then to take responsibility for decisions.

UNPREDICTABILITY OF COURSE OF ILLNESS

Many persons, including hospital staff, the client, and the family, ask variations of the question, "How long will I live?" The question is not rooted in curiosity as much as in our fears of dying and death.

Statistics are available for the length of living past diagnosis (Harris, 1990; Lemp, Payne, Neal, Temelso, & Rutherford, 1990, for example) but they tend to be less helpful to the individual than most realize. Statistics are based on tendencies within large groups. Means (averages), medians (half of a group are above the median; half below), modes (clusters of individuals on a certain score), and standard deviations (a measure of a range within a group) are descriptive of general tendencies in large groups, but not of individuals. As such, quoting statistics to an individual is likely to be misleading.

Those with AIDS-related experience will answer the question, "How long will I live?" by saying truthfully, "There's no way to know." All have seen patients who have died quickly and unexpectedly. One summer afternoon I met Angelo in his hospital room. He was talkative, anxious, and needy. My report described how quickly he could drain a caregiver with his many requests for information and his apparent obliviousness to the information provided. He was ill, but looked robust, and everything about him suggested a long course of illness. The next day, there was a staff meeting regarding the psychological issues around questions of time of death. At the end of the meeting, a "Code 99" called for a rescuscitation team. Angelo had died, suddenly and unexpectedly.

The contrary is also repeatedly seen. Jimmy, a former entertainer, had perhaps one of the longest courses of AIDS. He had multiple hospitalizations, an indwelling catheter, MAI and, later, dementia. I telephoned him during one of his hospitalizations, and he thanked me for visiting him that morning, when I had not. He told his psychiatrist, "I don't like you because I don't like anyone who dresses better than me." He made sure his nurses provided ample care. On Monday, he was mentally crisp, on Tuesday he was delirious. He hung on to life, and made everyone realize how alive he was, for many years.

For the HIV-positive person, the unpredictability of course of illness is another emotional burden, and a common psychotherapy theme (see Chapter 5).

In conclusion, although HIV is a condition with physical, emotional, spiritual, and other concerns, the client is first pulled into a highly complex medical subculture, which can be confusing and terrifying. With time to sort and understand information, the terror subsides and the work on the emotional and psychological aspects can begin. The psychotherapist working with the HIV-positive person must be conversant and comfortable with the medical aspects of this condition, and able to use this information to understand the client's emotional responses.

3
Sociopolitical Issues

AIDS, a constellation of medical conditions, is also a constellation of psychological, political, social, and, ultimately, economic issues unlike those provoked by any other condition.

- A gubernatorial candidate in New Jersey announces that he opposes classroom teaching by anyone with AIDS.
- A Catholic bishops organization rejects advocacy of condom use and urges only chastity as a preventive measure against AIDS.
- Child welfare systems are increasingly challenged by the growing number of HIV-infected mothers and babies. Yet, a newspaper headline notes drug treatment that could prevent infection is scarcer than ever for women (Diesenhouse, 1990).

This list continues to lengthen, so much that an international commentator wrote, "The third epidemic—of social, cultural, economic, and political reaction and response—threatens increasingly to overshadow and overwhelm the epidemics of HIV and AIDS" (Mann, 1989, p. 2). Perhaps we already are awash in the third epidemic, a tidal wave of sociopolitical concerns triggered by the earthquakes called morality and mortality.

Most can recall the societal responses to Legionnaire's Disease or Toxic Shock Syndrome, two medical conditions which struck a relatively small number of persons. People were appalled, and sympathetic to those affected. Demands were made for quick unraveling of those medical mysteries. The response to HIV has been markedly dissimilar. Fascination is replaced by disgust, sympathy with vilification.

What is different about AIDS? One obvious difference is the community's initial lack of empathy for the majority of those with HIV infection, persons already stigmatized for being "different." In some larger cities, gay men and women have achieved greater acceptance and political power. But, in many communities, openly gay lifestyles still are viewed with some, or a great deal of, discomfort. There is little sympathy anywhere for the intravenous drug user. They are seen as criminals, willing participants in a drug lifestyle, judged in moral terms by many. Also judged in moral terms are the means of becoming infected: sex, particularly anal sex, and use of contaminated needles. The moral judgments are often revealed in such comments as "innocent victims of AIDS," usually referring to children or those infected through transfusions. The others are guilty . . . of what? While AIDS has forced many religious groups to re-examine their theological convictions, most are careful not to appear to accept the lifestyles of most with AIDS (Steinfels, 1989, p. 5). The unsatisfying notion that "we love the sinner but hate the sin" still permeates many church statements without acknowledgment that not all agree on what is sin.

Unlike those with other illnesses, persons with AIDS are not generally seen as courageous and receive hardly a fraction of the sympathy reserved for those, say, with Alzheimer's Disease—even though persons no more seek out HIV than they do Alzheimer's. Many were infected at a time when nothing was known of HIV; most of those later infected do not have the psychological, cognitive, or other resources to incorporate knowledge about AIDS and use that to halt addictive drug-seeking behaviors. In any event, when have we as a society last been so angry with physically ill persons? Where has the compassion gone?

An analytic explanation is provided by Stevens and Muskin (1987) who suggest that lack of compassion for a PWA results from unconscious identification with that person, who represents loss of control of primitive impulses: "In order to protect themselves from the unconscious fear that they will be punished for the loss of impulse control they perceive in the AIDS patient, some people need to maintain the illusion that the AIDS victim is unlike them in any way" (p. 543). We unconsciously identify with the PWA, the authors suggest, then externalize the feared wishes to be bad or the fear that we have been bad in the past, and then "to avoid the seduction of these wishes, it is necessary to avoid the 'bad' patient" (p. 543). The authors note that the punishment for the perceived transgressions is seen as death, without appeal or hope of rescue, raising primitive childhood fears of annihilation. The PWA, who stimulates these fears, is feared and hated for bringing this disaster: "To survive, the individual needs to keep the AIDS patient at arm's length, both emotionally and physically" (p. 543). Moreover, the PWA "viewed as a devalued object by some people, may stimulate sexual fantasies involving the object or lead to seeking out the devalued object in reality. The shame and guilt aroused by such sexual fantasies as well as the fear that is evoked by the possibility of actualizing the fantasies may also create a barrier to the emergence of empathy" (p. 545).

Added to the morality issue is another unapproachable issue: mortality. AIDS was seen initially as an inevitably fatal illness. Now, it can be more acurately described as a chronic and sometimes life-threatening illness. With new prophylactic medicines and better treatment, HIV-infected persons are living longer. Nevertheless, because we are so uncomfortable with issues of death, we put emotional space between us and persons viewed as dying (see Becker's Pulitzer-prize winning *Denial of Death,* 1973, for an analysis of our terror of death).

Many see AIDS as someone else's problem. Areas outside New York and San Francisco see AIDS as the problem of those cities. That may have once been true, but by 1991 80% of new AIDS cases will be from outside those two cities (National Commission on AIDS, 1989). Gay AIDS-related organizations have been criticized for ignoring the interests of other HIV-infected persons, notably IVDUs and women. And many whites cannot see AIDS as their problem because many infected are persons of color.

The moral judgments and the "them, not us" view effectively preclude a clear vision of the current and future situations, as well as the determination to systematically, and systemically, plan for the future. Many have an inkling that a disaster is at hand, but most believe it will happen elsewhere or, at the very least, to someone else.

In the United States, plenty of warnings have been voiced, and most have been ignored. In June 1988 The Presidential Commission on the Human Immunodeficiency Virus Epidemic issued its report, a humane and wide-ranging document. Some 600 recommendations were made, including 20 which form the framework of a "comprehensive national strategy" (p. xvii) to manage the epidemic. These recommendations include:

- Early detection, with more widespread availability of HIV tests.
- Consideration of HIV infection as a disability under federal and state law.
- More stringent protection in federal and state law for privacy, with significant penalties for violations.
- Prevention and treatment of IV drug abuse as a top national priority.
- Examination of "more equitable and cost-effective financing of care" (p. xvii).
- Development and implementation of age-appropriate education programs from kindergarten through grade 12.
- Aggressive attention to the problems of teenagers that place them at risk.

Few of these have been acted upon and the report itself is now difficult to find. About 18 months later, in December 1989, the National Commission on Acquired Immune Deficiency Syndrome issued its first report, outlining four "clear and alarming" (p. 2) messages heard in testimony from experts:

- A dangerous complacency exists and may be growing regarding AIDS.
- The 1990s will be "much worse" (p. 2) than the 1980s when the epidemic

will reach crisis proportions among the young, poor, women, and in minority communities.
- Links between HIV infection and drug use must be addressed in a national drug strategy.
- No national plan exists to help already faltering health care systems deal with HIV.

The commission's report described the numbers of affected persons involved, and noted that "a series of problems have resulted in a health care system singularly unresponsive to the needs of HIV infected people" (p. 4). Some, with no doctor, clinic, or means of payment, have only one doorway to medical care, that of the emergency room. Further, there still remains the question of who will pay for the many with AIDS in the 1990s. "The belief that Medicaid will pay for the health care needs of the growing number of low income people with HIV infection and AIDS is, as one expert witness told the Commission, a 'Medicaid fantasy' " (p. 4).

The commission delineated four areas of attention:

1. Recognition that a crisis exists and will require significant changes in how we think about the health care system.
2. Creation of a flexible and patient-oriented comprehensive care system, which will link hospital, ambulatory, residential, and home care. Primary care physicians will need financial, social, and institutional support.
3. Consideration of creation of regional care centers, to provide backup and consultation to community-based care providers.
4. Creation of centers that would treat those with HIV infection and drug addiction.

In addition, 1990s public policy debate regarding HIV will include these issues:

- Preventing or condoning?

Within this area is broad discourse focused on several issues, including provision of clean needles to addicts, condoms to prisoners, and AIDS-related sexual education to adolescents. On one hand are the persons who claim these activities take reality into account, and serve to prevent HIV transmission. On the other hand are those who say these activities condone and, perhaps, even encourage illegal or immoral behavior.

The sociopolitical tension around these issues was illustrated in New York City, where a new mayor closed a city-run needle exchange program just after the outgoing city health commissioner reported such programs "can be an effective 'bridge to treatment' for IV drug users" (New York City Department of Health, 1989, unnumbered page). Proponents of such programs argue that no evidence exists that these programs encourage intravenous drug use (Watters et al., 1990, for example).

Similar debates are occurring regarding prisoners' access to condoms when sexual activity is not allowed, and provision of HIV-related information and condoms to teenagers. Proponents say sexual activity occurs, and condoms would prevent spread of HIV. Opponents say this would encourage sexual behavior that is not permitted or acceptable.

• Balancing the rights of individuals.

Discussions in this area usually involve the rights of an HIV-infected person or one suspected of infection (even without reason). Should rapists be tested for HIV? How does one balance peace-of-mind to victims versus the privacy rights of those accused or convicted of crimes? (This has already been a topic on the television show, "L.A. Law.")

Should the names of HIV-infected persons be reported to public health agencies, and their sex- or needle-sharing partners traced and notified? Proponents say early detection may prolong life. Opponents say this would violate the privacy rights of AIDS patients (Lambert, 1989).

It is unlikely that our clients will raise these issues in psychotherapy sessions. Many of these issues—that they come up at all, that we ignore them or debate them interminably—have to do with the societal psyche. They affect us all.

COMMUNITY RESOURCES

Communities' feelings about persons who may be HIV infected are likely to be reflected in the services available. If a community is ambivalent, services may have a mix of good and poor aspects. If the community is hostile, poor or no services may be available, requiring the client to travel to obtain specialized services.

At least one research report indicates that a patient's search for AIDS specialty centers is worth the effort. Bennett et al. (1989) found that hospitals that had a high level of experience with AIDS patients had lower rates of mortality due to PCP compared to rates in hospitals with less AIDS experience.

In choosing a physician to treat HIV-related conditions, the rule of thumb should be the same as in finding a surgeon: Hire one with experience in the specialty. However, practice varies even in the field of AIDS, therefore other factors need to be considered. These include:

• Is the physician's practice consonant with the client's wishes about treatment?

Even among AIDS specialists there is a wide range of practice—from the creative use of medications not yet federally approved for AIDS patients, to a very conservative "by the book" practice that discourages prescription of nonapproved drugs as well as the patient's obtaining drugs via buyer's clubs or grey markets. A practitioner in upstate New York, for example, might tell a gathering that his medical practice prescribed aerosolized pentamadine for PCP prophylaxis 2 years before it was approved for that use. Even within a large city, the patient is subjected to the vagaries of medical practice. One medical center's AIDS practitioners may depend on Dapsone for PCP prophylaxis, while another's, just a mile down a main road, may prefer Bactrim. Each group of doctors is practicing good medicine, based on its best hunches and readings of the research, and one treatment's superiority may emerge only after some time, if at all.

A large part of healing, however, comes from a consonance between physician and patient. The patient should seek one with a similar treatment philosophy.

- Does the physician provide access or facilitate access to drug trials? Some doctors, notably those in specialized AIDS services, participate in investigational studies. Others may refer their patients to these studies. Does the physician facilitate such participation?
- Is the physician comfortable with the patient's lifestyle, be it gay, bisexual, heterosexual, or drug dependent?
- Is the office staff comfortable with the patient? While infection control measures must be taken when there is possibility of contact with bodily fluids, do nurses or physician's assistants wear gowns, masks, or gloves for interviews?
- Is confidentiality assured?

Other community resources which may be important to the client include, obviously, mental health services, either in hospital, community, or private practice settings. Because of the likelihood of HIV-related psychiatric manifestations, access to a psychiatrist familiar with HIV illness and psychopharmacology is necessary. Often lacking, in addition, is access to spiritual resources: ministers, rabbis, or others who can relate to an HIV-positive person without communicating potentially damaging judgments.

SPECIAL NEEDS OF WOMEN

Because of already-existing discrimination against women, the HIV-positive woman, whose psychosocial situation can be extremely complex, is likely to be severely underserved.

A woman is likely to have been infected either by heterosexual transmission or by intravenous drug use. She may have survived her spouse or partner who has died of AIDS, and is caring for one or several children. Other family members, such as the woman's parents, may be involved as caregivers.

The HIV-positive woman faces great hostility from both the public and professionals. Her HIV status may be viewed as an indication of promiscuity or consort with a repugnant sex partner. If drug use was involved and, especially, if it is continuing, service providers may be very angry and critical, perceiving her as a neglectful mother who continues to jeopardize her children. However, little consideration is given to the psychological issues of drug dependence and the shortage of drug-abuse treatment and other social services available to women, including pregnant women and mothers.

If a woman who is potentially or actually HIV-positive is pregnant or considering pregnancy, several other issues come into play. Special counseling is needed to explain the possibility of HIV transmission to the child and, if the woman is pregnant, her options regarding abortion or bringing the fetus to term.

An especially crucial women's issue, with some thorny medical ethics and civil rights considerations, is how HIV-related medical treatment differs for a pregnant woman, compared to that for a non-pregnant woman or a man. A case in point is the use of zidovudine—many physicians will not treat pregnant HIV-positive women with zidovudine, which is suspected of being injurious to a fetus. Regarding immediate prophylactic use of zidovudine after suspected occupational exposure to HIV, Gelberding (1990), in response to a question, said her facility did not offer the prophylaxis to women who are pregnant or suspected of being pregnant. In making these decisions, medical professionals and institutions appear to hold the right of the fetus superior to the woman's right to the best medical treatment available. Some would question that stance, and argue that the woman has the right to be offered prompt and state-of-the-art treatment, allowing her to make an informed decision. The fetus-versus-mother issue has been raised by Annas (1987) and Kolder, Gallagher, and Parsons (1987) in non-HIV contexts.

The mother who faces hospitalization for HIV-related illness and does not have dependable caregivers for her children may attempt to postpone hospitalization. Or, she may be reluctant to discuss that situation, fearing service providers will report possible neglect to a child welfare agency. The client fears that her family will be injured, and that she will be further stigmatized. Furthermore, service providers may be angry with being faced with a common dilemma: Forced by law to report the situation to an inadequate and unsympathetic agency, the professional realizes the relationship with the client is jeopardized for little benefit to the children. In sum, social service providers find cases involving women to be much more problematic, due to the lack of family services and the need for case management that extends to the children's needs.

Medical services for women, too, are more complicated. Special needs include such specialty doctors such as gynecologists, obstetricians, and nurses who are sympathetic and supportive. New mothers must have access to pediatricians who understand the mechanics of in utero HIV transmission and, if the child is HIV-positive, are able to treat the condition.

FINANCIAL ISSUES

Any chronic illness represents a drain on personal resources. AIDS as a chronic illness has several complexities which require careful research and planning. The first step is a complete financial assessment, according to Thomas Watson, a hospital resource coordinator who has worked with a spectrum of clients over 20 years (personal communication, December 1989). This assessment should respond to the question, "How will I live?" and should inventory available funds, insurance, Social Security, and other available entitlements, and expenses such as rent or mortgage, medical expenses, and other living expenses. Other factors must also be taken into account: extent of medical insurance coverage, the quality of available public and Medicaid-funded medical care, and the willingness of the patient's private physician to take Medicaid payments.

Employment

Important to most clients is the ability to continue working. Many symptomatic HIV-positive persons, even those with a diagnosis of AIDS, are able to continue employment, especially if the jobs are not physically taxing. The client may want to continue to work for the feelings of well-being, usefulness, camaraderie and other intangible as well as tangible benefits of employment.

If the client is beginning to consider leaving work, the first step is to check the employee benefits, to determine what entitlements exist upon leaving, Watson urges.

A person will be eligible for Social Security Disability only if he or she is judged unable to work and has worked "on the books" (that is, with taxes deducted and records kept) and paid into Social Security for 5 of the past 10 years. If found eligible, no payment will be made for the first 5 months of disability. The payment for the 6th month will arrive at the beginning of the 7th month. Some states will provide disability payments until the federal monies begin; others do not. The federal payment schedule is clearly defined. More money is provided to younger persons, and more is provided to those who had higher earnings, but the payments are meager compared to regular wages.

If a person is disabled and has not worked "on the books" or paid into Social Security, he or she may be eligible for Supplementary Security Income (SSI) if current assets are less than $2,000. Along with SSI, Medicaid benefits are dispensed by most states, subject to their regulations. Because these regulations vary, the safe approach is to check with the local office that dispenses these benefits.

It is recommended that the employer's medical insurance benefits be scrutinized. If that insurance pays for doctor and hospital bills but not for prescriptions, the costs of those pharmaceuticals may severely strain the budget. While costs for some of the prophylactic medications (such as zidovudine) are declining, use of several medications can cost upwards of $10,000 annually. Moreover, even if someone has a policy that pays for prescriptions, an insurance company may decline to reimburse for drugs prescribed for an HIV-related condition if the federal government has not approved them for that use. Such was the case with pentamidine, which for some time was prescribed but not approved for prophylactic use. Some states have programs that pay for prophylactic medications, notably zidovudine, which should be investigated. Otherwise, without insurance coverage or state aid, the client may have to pay for the medication "out of pocket."

These out-of-pocket expenses may also include costs for pharmaceuticals purchased through buying clubs. In several metropolitan areas, PWA advocacy groups have set up organizations to help purchase and, in some cases, smuggle unapproved drugs from other countries. While the clubs reduce costs, the expenses still may be high.

Other out-of-pocket costs may include: payments to psychotherapists, if not covered by the employer's policy or if the annual limit is exceeded; extra payments to physicians and other health professionals not enrolled in "preferred provider" programs offered by some policies; home-care expenses and other costs above what private insurers reimburse.

Faced with these and other expenses, an HIV-positive person who is becoming disabled may eventually face a hard choice: stay working, using the employer's health policy and spending savings (if any exist), or leave work, spending savings if required and going on Social Security and receiving Medicaid. The disadvantages of Medicaid coverage include many physicians' refusal to take Medicaid's typically low reimbursement, and possible poor quality of care in public hospitals or "house service" wards in private hospitals, relative to private patient care. Some psychotherapists are reimbursed poorly or not at all by Medicaid.

Some HIV-positive persons now prepare years in advance for sickness and possible need for Medicaid by distributing savings and property to friends and relatives. Watson suggests that a person "enjoy life" before becoming disabled. This may include spending some savings on travel, relatives, and friends. Once one applies for disability, the government may see such spending as a way to evade savings ceilings. Some persons choose to work "off the books" (without tax records) and continue to receive Medicaid benefits, although this is illegal. Another option, available to a high-functioning patient who is asymptomatic, is employment in a company that has very good group benefits, with the intent of staying there through the chronic illness. Even if the illness forces departure from the job, the benefits may be continued, although paid for by the client (or Medicaid) through a plan called COBRA (which stands for Consolidated Omnibus Budget Reconciliation Act, which contains the provision for this option). No one should depart a job for unemployment without studying the COBRA options. Others seek part-time work with temporary agencies that offer insurance benefits.

Life Insurance

When an individual now applies for a life insurance policy, it is unlikely that a policy will be written without an HIV test. Insurance applications ask about HIV status, and payments may be refused upon a finding that a person died of HIV-related illness which was denied upon application.

However, several options remain. One is to seek employment at a company that offers group insurance as an automatic benefit. Some may be able to obtain group-term insurance through professional groups, college alumni organizations, credit card memberships, and other clubs and associations.

Discrimination

Among the problems faced by HIV-positive persons is discrimination based on their condition. No legal recourse based on federal statutes has been available. However, in July 1990 Congress passed and the President signed the Americans with Disabilities Act, drafted to bar discrimination against disabled persons, including persons with AIDS, in the workplace and in public accommodations, transportation and telephone services. The law will require employers to make reasonable accomodations to allow handicapped workers to continue employment, and would bar hiring discrimination against disabled persons. Different aspects of the law will take effect at different times, and regulations regarding enforcement and penalties for violations may not be completed until late 1991.

Best Natural Resource: "Family"

It is almost simplistic to note that the client's best natural resource is "family," not only blood relatives but also any friends who have a relationship with the HIV-positive person. The effect of failure to enlist family resources can be drastic. But if the client is estranged from family and wants no reconciliation, there may be little a therapist can do. However, few persons are so solitary as to not have a friend, neighbor, lover, spouse, or sibling available for helping.

Several uses of family resources are possible:

1. As leverage toward therapy goals.

If, for example, a therapy goal is compliance, caregivers may be able to aid the client toward improved compliance. Familiarity with family dynamics may also be useful because caregivers may be surreptitiously sabotaging compliance, or the client may be behaving in reaction to perceived feelings of caregivers.

2. For improvement in quality of client care, either at home or during hospitalization.

Social support is useful, but trained social support is more useful. With some training, family members may be able to provide better home care and may be more attuned to incipient emergencies. Caregivers also can, for an ill family member, learn to monitor such hospital and home care as medications, which are sometimes erroneously given.

3. For a decreased level of tension.

If a client has an alternative lifestyle that is rejected by the primary family, there may be tension between the client's family of origin and his or her new family (lovers, friends). An intervention with family members may be to acquaint them with the effects of the continuing struggle on the patient, and seek a truce, if not a resolution.

Some may say that these social, political and financial issues are not the stuff of psychotherapy, and are better discussed at political meetings or with resource counselors. Yet, they are part of the context which affect our HIV-positive clients and our communities, as well. To fail to understand these issues is to fail to understand the sociopolitical context in which our HIV-positive clients live.

PART 2

THE WORK OF PSYCHOTHERAPY

4
Assessment of
the Therapeutic Contract

The psychotherapeutic relationship with an HIV-positive person finds its direction with a vigilant intake assessment.

Competent but leisurely intake assessments done over many sessions well suit the work with a stable client or one contemplating long-term therapy. What is different about the work with an HIV-positive client is that circumstances, already potentially quite complex, can quickly change. Therefore, the assessment of an HIV-positive person should cover more ground more rapidly. This is especially true if the client already is diagnosed with AIDS.

This full view of the client's current psychological, medical, and social situation provides a base of knowledge useful in two ways. First, the information helps the therapist decide if the "fit" is right—whether the therapist can provide what is needed and offer a therapeutic contract or, instead, make a timely referral. Second, the assessment provides a baseline against which psychological, cognitive, and other medical changes are gauged. These changes, which can come often, must always be noted and sometimes acted upon. (See "Therapist's Monitoring Function," Chapter 6.)

As I was writing the preceeding paragraphs, I took a phone call that notified me that a hospital patient had died. This young man, 30, was severely limited by a personality disorder. Hospitalized up to three weeks ago for PCP, he was a difficult patient, demanding that staff instantly meet his needs. He told me a wildly contradictory story that changed even during the telling. He had a girl friend; he didn't. He was a professional gambler; no, he was a state employee. He was agitated, unpleasant, manipulative, and he fled the hospital the moment he felt able. He returned, however. Yesterday, he found himself

43

in a Manhattan hospital's emergency room and he announced he was there to die. He was admitted, and he died within hours. Other examples abound. One week two of my outpatients were fit and well. The following Monday, both were hospitalized—one for sepsis and the other for a gastric bleed.

A full-ranging assessment is important also because the illness's unpredictability affects the psychosocial environment. One patient's caregiver fled in panic as the patient entered the Intensive Care Unit. The caregiver was not seen again. The psychotherapist must be prepared for these occurrences, as well as to witness many caregivers' heroisms. Among the tenderest of my memories is that of a man hospitalized in a ward specifically for New York state prisoners with AIDS. He was crying because a friend, another prisoner, had died that morning of AIDS. He told me, "I spent three days at his bedside, holding his hand."

INTAKE ASSESSMENT

The following outline for the initial intake is suggested:

Medical condition. A sweeping view of the client's current health status is required. The following information should be among that gathered:

- Current status: HIV-positive, ARC, or AIDS? Even given the shortcomings of the CDC criteria, this indicates the patient's medical situation and affects medical care, the possibility of entitlements and, of course, the therapeutic contract.
- HIV-related illnesses (and other recent illnesses) that have occurred, when, and the shortterm and lasting effects.
- Name of treating physician and his or her expertise. Names of other professional caregivers: dentist, ophthalmologist, respiratory therapist, occupational therapist, nutritionist or dietician, social workers, and their affiliations.
- The name of the client's hospital or clinic. Is the client treated in another city? Why? Research indicates clients have a better chance of in-hospital survival if they are treated in a hospital with more AIDS experience (Bennett et al., 1989). Depending on geography, specialized units may not be available. Persons may commute to specialty hospitals either for better care or because of fear of disclosure locally. Certainly the patient's attending physician should have AIDS-related expertise. The choice of caregiver may provide information about the patient's motivation.
- Prescribed medications currently used, and those that were tried and found to be ineffective or with serious side effects. These include medications for prophylaxis, such as zidovudine and aerosolized pentamidine. Are any psychiatric medications? Sometimes antidepressants are used for pain, and the

patient is not told the medication is actually an antidepressant. Those treated by sophisticated practitioners sometimes also receive antidepressants, antipsychotics or amphetamines for effects of AIDS dementia complex.

- Reasons for not using commonly used prophylactic medications, such as zidovudine. Here it may be useful to explore the client's motivations and beliefs regarding prophylactic medication. Zidovudine has been found to be useful to some who are HIV-positive but asymptomatic, and advocacy groups have affirmed this. Some persons have tried it and have suffered massive declines of white blood cells, which make this treatment unwise. Others, however, have beliefs that the medication poisons the system. Extreme beliefs should be noted and explored.
- Response to treatment, generally.
- Is the patient receiving home-based medical care? Among the new medical technologies available is infusion therapy for those able to receive certain medications at home. DHPG, for CMV retinitis, can be provided by a home nursing agency, as can total parenteral nutrition for those suffering from wasting syndrome. These home therapies need not limit the patient's independence; there are portable, unobtrusive pumps, and many intravenous medications can be provided at night and disconnected in the morning.

Patient's knowledge about medical condition.

- How much does the client know about his or her medical condition? If he or she is vague or there is a lack of knowledge, why? Are there pockets of lack of knowledge? These may indicate psychological trouble areas.
- The client's beliefs or delusions about HIV generally, his or her HIV status, and stated willingness and ability to survive.
- Degree of denial and realism, the nature of his or her fighting spirit.

Observe the consonance between medical condition and degree of denial. If the client is vague or unsophisticated, or seems impaired, the clinician should obtain a two-way waiver of confidentiality from the client, enabling a dialog between you and other professional caregivers.

Cognitive functioning.

AIDS-related dementia is likely to affect the majority of AIDS patients. A preliminary screening for cognitive dysfunction is necessary (see Chapter 7 for an extended discussion of neuropsychological effects of HIV).

A nonintrusive introduction into this area can be the simple question, "How has your memory been lately?" Many patients will readily admit to some memory lapses, if they occur. Even if the client says he or she is fine, follow by saying, "Let me ask a few quick questions to test your memory." One guide to such screening is Berg, Franzen, and Wedding's (1987) *Screening for Brain Impairment: A Manual for Mental Health Practice.* Others suggest use of the mental status exam described by Mueller (1984) or, if signs of dementia are more obvious, the Blessed Dementia Scale (Blessed, Tomlinson, & Roth, 1968).

Psychiatric/psychological history and current workup.

A study of 207 persons who sought free HIV-antibody testing at a major medical center found a high percentage of men and women had current mood disorders while a high percentage of women had current alcohol and nonintravenous substance abuse diagnoses, compared to a community sample. Moreover, compared to a control community sample, there were much higher rates of mood disorders and nonalcohol substance dependence in both men and women and alcohol dependence in women who sought testing. In another setting, a man who sought psychotherapy had been prescribed Xanax for a panic disorder. But he never was asked about voices, which he had heard since his teenage years in a detention center. These illustrate the need for taking histories during the assessment process. The following should be included:

- Diagnostic workups for Axis I and II disorders. If a mood disorder is indicated, determine onset and assess the possibility that it may be organic and HIV-related (see Chapter 6 for additional information). Ask specifically about suicidal ideation and intent (see Chapter 6). Researchers found that 14 of 49 seropositive persons reported suicidal ideation at time of HIV testing; of 252 seronegative persons, 77 (30.6%) reported suicidal ideation at time of testing (Perry, Jacobsberg, & Fishman, 1990).
- Previous history with mental health professionals. You may need to specify such professions as pastoral counselors, psychologists or psychiatrists (many confuse these two), or program counselors, usually taken to mean substance abuse counselors.
- Participation, current or past, in Narcotics Anonymous (NA), Alcoholics Anonymous (AA), Positives Anonymous (for HIV-positive persons), Sex Anonymous, or other 12-step programs. One example of an obscure program based on 12-step principles is Courage, an orthodox Catholic program that encourages celibacy among gay men and women.
- Use of psychiatric medication, either prescribed or from street purchases. Usually it helps to list street drugs commonly used in your community. I will say, "Have you ever taken Librium (pause for response), Valium (pause . . .)," and so on with Xanax, Thorazine, Haldol, Navane, Stelazine. I also add "or any drugs with names like these?" Gay men, too, should be asked about street purchases.

History of substance use and abuse.

- Any experience with alcohol, heroin, cocaine, other drugs, or any combination of drugs (e.g., cocaine and heroin, "speedballing"). Were they taken by nose or by needle? How much and how often?

- Has usage changed since knowledge of HIV diagnosis? Many drug-using persons attempt to assuage their psychological distress with increased use of street drugs.
- Is the person enrolled in a drug treatment program, or does he or she attend NA or AA meetings? If in a methadone program, what was the starting dosage and what is the current dosage? Who is the physician and counselor there? Can you speak with them? Drug treatment counselors can be sources of information as well as sources of leverage with the patient. Patients tend to have longstanding relationships with their counselors. If there are complaints about the relationship, or no relationship, that may predict the client's response to you.

Psychosocial background.

- Names and positions of caregivers. Does the client have two families—one of blood relatives and another of affiliation? The affiliative family may be one of gay men or women, or one of a drug subculture, or simply a family that has taken the client in during times of difficulty.
- Are the relatives supportive or rejecting? If absent, why?
- Who will make treatment decisions for the patient if incapacitation occurs? Are these the caregivers or different persons, and why?
- Is the relationship of client and caregivers stable and committed? Are the caregivers healthy or are they anticipating debilitation? If caregivers are physically ill, or elderly, the patient may not trust that they can provide adequate longterm care.
- If there is social isolation, what is the cause? Is there schizoidal process, rigid family beliefs?
- Who else can be counted on in an emergency?
- Whom should you contact in any emergency?
- What should you do if the client misses an appointment and you cannot reach him or her? Is there someone you can call to find if there is something wrong? Or is the client socially isolated? What arrangements can be made to ensure the safety, over the long term, of a socially isolated client? One therapist told a slightly demented client who lived alone that the police would be called if the client failed to appear for an appointment and did not call within eight hours to explain.
- Can the caregivers be organized to care for the patient?

Sexual functioning, past and current.

- Straight, gay, or bisexual?
- Number of partners; serial monogamy, casual sex, monogamy.
- Type of sex preferred? Anal, oral? Receptive?
- Has this changed since diagnosis or opportunistic infection?
- Currently sexually active?

- Practicing safer sex?
- Any unwanted sexual occurrences? This question encompasses incest, fondling, and/or rape. It is remarkable the number of gay men and women who report unwanted childhood sexual experiences.
- If the client is gay, ask when he or she first recognized feelings of homosexuality.

This provides an opening question for sexual history. An exploration of this aspect of the client's life is in order, as well as an inquiry into the understanding of the etiology of homosexuality, and its personal and social consequences.

The answers to these questions accomplish the following: First, they help establish a baseline against which the therapist can judge such things as (a) medical changes and emergencies, (b) changes in cognitive or social functioning, and (c) new or exacerbated dysfunctions in the client's support system.

Second, and as important, these questions provide data by which the clinician can gauge what the psychotherapeutic contract may entail. The therapist may at some point be asked by the client or required by circumstances to take more of a case-management role (see Chapter 8); many patients may have a stable support system or a companion that will provide case management. But others will not, or relationships change; caregivers can get ill. With a good initial assessment, you can discern what the client's needs are likely to be, and decide whether you can comfortably work with those needs.

THE THERAPEUTIC CONTRACT

With knowledge of the basic course of HIV-related illnesses and a vigilant intake, the psychotherapist has important information to help anticipate issues that may arise during the psychotherapy. The information helps the therapist to consider two issues: What type of therapeutic contract will be effective? And, can the therapist provide that type of contract?

The quick and incomplete response to the first question is that the contract will be based in large part on the therapist's training within a specific paradigm. While this is true, the response is more complete if two other aspects are added: the therapist's conception of "caring" and "therapeutic relationship" and the professional flexibility within that paradigm to respond to changing needs.

As noted earlier, movement along a continuum of psychotherapeutic care is suggested—ranging from encouragement of exploration to interpersonal dialogues to, if necessary and mutually agreed upon, case management. The professional should feel free, within one's competence, to respond therapeutically to the ever-changing situations caused by HIV-related chronicity.

The therapist who adheres rigidly to the mechanics of the paradigm—to the "frame"—will likely be unable to serve fully the HIV-positive person. Difficulties will arise, first, because the HIV-positive person probably does not fit into neatly described diagnostic or other categories. Second, the frame may be perceived as societal rules that in different degrees were used to denigrate the client and instill self-loathing.

One is not asked to throw away the book. But one is asked if the book has a response to the changing human needs of this very distressed population. For example, it is not suggested that the therapist should collude with circumvention of the therapy hour by way of lengthy phone calls. The appropriate response is, as always: "Is there a crisis? What crisis intervention can be provided? Let's meet soon to discuss this." But what if the patient is bedridden and a face-to-face meeting is impossible? Do we forgo therapy?

OTHER PSYCHOTHERAPEUTIC CONSIDERATIONS

As we assess the contract, other issues to be explored include:

Missed Appointments

One of the discouraging aspects of psychotherapy with PWAs is missed appointments. The reasons given include fatigue or other physical symptoms, bad weather or transportation problems. This presents problems for private practitioners who are used to compliant patients and filled hours. If Medicaid is paying, the missed appointment also represents lost income.

The real reasons for missed appointments should be investigated, and their significance addressed. If the client clearly prefers less-frequent meetings, can this schedule be negotiated to both parties' satisfaction? Can therapy goals be met if meetings are less frequent?

If a person cancels because of genuine problems, such as physical incapacitation, can some accommodation be made that will allow the relationship to continue? If geography and transportation are not too difficult, can the therapist make a "house call?" Is telephone therapy appropriate with a bedridden patient?

Sandy, who has had AIDS more than 2 years, wants to be seen only every 2 or 3 weeks. He explains, "I don't have much energy, and anyway I've got the situation pretty much in control. I just need time to sound off every now and then. It's really my friends who have the problems, not me."

Should the response be, "No, I really need to see you weekly if we are to make any progress." Or is an irregular program acceptable?

Duty to Warn of Threat of Infection

Raymond, an HIV-positive 25-year-old with a history of hearing voices, is a former intravenous drug user currently on methadone and an antidepressant. He has been in psychotherapy before and, one therapist learned later, was actually seeing two practitioners concurrently. Because of his experience with therapy and drug programs as well as a genuine native intelligence, Raymond was well-attuned to his feelings and insightful. Yet, he continued antisocial acts, and one day reported that he reinitiated a sexual relationship with a former sweetheart, and had unprotected sex. Told he must use condoms, Raymond responded, "I didn't use one the first time; she'll start asking questions if I start now."

In this case, the therapist concluded that Raymond was unlikely to protect the woman against HIV infection, but the woman's name was not known to the therapist and she could not be warned. But even if the woman's name was known, what are the psychotherapist's responsibilities?

Initially, the clinician will likely have to deal with his or her own intense feelings regarding the situation. Adler and Beckett (1989) describe the case of a sexually impulsive HIV-positive woman who had unprotected sex, and the reactions of the therapist. They note the force of projective identification, the necessity for the therapist to contain his or her feelings, and interpretation to the client of the meaning of the experience. In this case, the therapist elected to delay confronting and driving away the client.

But after feelings are contained, considerations of responsibility must follow. In professional training, the decision in *Tarasoff v. Regents of the University of California* (1976) is often cited as indicative of the therapist's responsibility to warn of danger, despite confidentiality. In that decision, the Supreme Court of California said that there is a responsibility to warn of foreseeable harm if the party has a special relationship to the dangerous person or potential victim. The court determined that the therapist–client relationship was special and the therapist had a sufficient relationship with this client to create a duty to warn a potential victim.

With HIV specifically, no courts or professional groups have issued rulings or guidelines. Some states have laws allowing disclosure but none require warnings of danger. The therapist, faced with a client who may infect another person with HIV, has no solid basis upon which to resolve the dilemma.

North and Rothenberg (1990) argue that there is no tension between confidentiality and the duty to warn, that "professions have always allowed for exceptions to absolute confidentiality" (p. 134). They suggest a case-by-case determination based on a risk–benefit assessment that includes these factors: foreseeability of harm, including assessment of the client's veracity; knowledge of the potential victim's identity; consideration whether a warning will make a difference; consideration of the potential victim's other risk behaviors; community standards of moral blame and public policy; confidentiality laws; other costs; and potential for violence to the patient. While North and Rothenberg's (1990) article focused on the dilemma of a physician, their arguments assume no medical information not available to sophisticated psychotherapists. Their risk–benefit suggestions, however, beg the question of the liability of a therapist if insufficient or erroneous information is factored into the equation.

For the psychotherapist, the following suggestions are offered, with the knowledge that they too will be controversial and are hardly the final words on the matter:

- The therapist should immediately take a prevention stance. The client's knowledge regarding safer sex and drug use practices must be assessed and augmented. Both skills—such as condom use and drug paraphernalia cleaning—and the knowledge of potential danger to the partner should be stressed.
- A session involving the partner should be suggested, not for exploration of psychopathology or systems therapy, but for skills assessment and training for both persons. This session may also provide information regarding the potential victim's risks.
- If the client indicates unsafe practices will continue, the practitioner should warn the client's partner, if that person is known. This should occur only after the following: the danger is clearly articulated to the client, the client again states opposition to safer practices and an intent to continue the unsafe practice, and the therapist states that he or she believes the responsibility to warn someone in danger overrides confidentiality. While this risks severing the therapeutic relationship, it appears by now that the therapist has no leverage over the client's patently dangerous behaviors. Given this, the therapist cannot overlook unsafe practice while waiting for the therapeutic bond to become firm.
- The case should be discussed with supervisors and colleagues and exhaustively documented.
- If it occurs, the meeting with the infected person's partner should be factual, with emphasis on the mechanics of transmission, the utility of HIV testing, and a statement that there is no clear knowledge, without HIV testing, that infection has occurred.

Family Concerns

No matter how calm they may appear, family, friends, and lovers of persons with AIDS are themselves anxious as they face the decline of a family member. Their concerns affect and may demoralize the patient. For instance, a familiar familial theme is the patient is not doing enough to care for himself or herself. This often is expressed in efforts to make the sick person eat, even though many patients suffer from AIDS-related anorexia that may be, in some, impossible to overcome. Family members become angry when the PWA by not eating appears to reject their efforts. They attribute that to a lack of will and a rejection of their caring, when in fact the PWA may be suffering from a reaction to drug treatment, or from AIDS-related anorexia or wasting.

Another family issue is caregiver fatigue, which sometimes occurs during a lengthy hospitalization. The client may perceive caregivers' fatigue, and interpret that as their desire that he or she die. The caregivers, on the other hand, may feel guilty regarding their "burnout" and anticipatory separations and bereavement.

In these cases and many others, the therapist may organize family therapy sessions to correct the perceptual disortions, normalize caregivers' feelings, and suggest concrete helps such as hiring home attendants.

COUNTERTHERAPEUTIC BEHAVIORS

Many techniques are attempted with HIV-positive persons, and many awkward and useless things are said, out of ignorance or awkwardness. Some of these include:

Exhortation. All have witnessed or heard about counselors whose intervention armamentarium has only one tool—exhortation or, less politely put, haranguing. Imagine yourself in hospital "pajamas" with your backside showing, and someone flying into your room with the following: "Mr. Smith, you really must take the morning dose of medication. That is my recommendation. It is for your own good. You need to take it." The exhortation fills the gap where relationship, understanding, and dialogue should be. When the urge to exhort makes itself known, explore the frustration or shortcoming in the relationship that it evidences.

False optimism. One counselor, upon seeing a very sick patient, immediately began saying, "Don't worry. Everything will be all right" and similar sentiments. This does nothing to alleviate the client's worries, which may be firmly based in his or her situation. These phrases are used to calm the anxieties of the speaker, rather than the client.

Certain phrases. Many things are said in haste and thoughtlessly by those who are frustrated or impatient with clients who tap feelings of impotence. These unhelpful phrases include:

- "We will all die sometime." Indeed, but most persons are not facing untimely deaths, or the anxieties that come with knowing they are likely to die within the next few years, if not the next few months. One patient, in response, said, "Yes, but sometime is likely to be sooner for me." Where does one go therapeutically from there?
- "You have a fatal illness and you need to begin preparation." This is the

typical thoughtless remark that reveals a failure to consider the defenses of the patient. A variation of this was actually said by a mental health professional, and the patient's response was, "If you don't get out of my room, I'll kill you first."

Rather than fill an awkward moment or quell anxiety with a "filler" sentence or two, a clinician may allow silence, and find feelings expressed therein. Usually the client knows that little can be said, and appreciates the clinician's recognition of that. Those silent moments may be the start of the therapeutic relationship.

5
Psychotherapy Goals and Themes

Are the goals and themes of HIV-related psychotherapy different from those in other psychotherapies?

Some would say no, arguing that the same concerns are voiced and the same dynamics revealed and interpreted—feelings and concerns regarding loss and abandonment, family and social issues, and life goals and disappointments. One analytically trained therapist said AIDS is rarely specifically discussed in her group of HIV-positive persons, but group members spend time crying together.

Others would argue that the goals and themes of HIV-related psychotherapy are qualitatively different in many ways. For one, the content—the thoughts and emotions, and their expressions—are products of the knowledge that one's life is likely foreshortened and will be more difficult physically and emotionally than one ever imagined. Also, themes and goals such as coming to terms and living with many uncertainties *are* different and directly related to the existential realities of HIV infection. Clients not faced with AIDS or other physical illnesses may discuss issues of quality of life counterposed with nonlife, but they do so without the sense of imminence and sharp urgency that HIV illness imposes. This sense was expressed by one PWA, in reaction to someone's awkward comment that "We will all die sometime." He said, "Yes, but sometime is likely to be sooner for me." Another client said it this way, "HIV is the finger on the fast-forward button."

This imminence—be it a matter of months or years—is the foundation of HIV-related psychotherapy. Thus, even if some, if not all, psychotherapeutic goals and themes are expressed in other psychotherapies, with HIV-infection they are experienced as more urgent: Many with AIDS have seen friends and acquaintances die, and many, at some point, experience their own lives as foreshortened. The chronic illness and the concerns it brings are not dreamy abstracts but difficult realities experienced up close.

Making a list is always hazardous because readers may interpret it as an attempt to homogenize psychotherapeutic content. Here the intent is to prepare the practitioner for what may emerge, acknowledging that the expressions will be personal and unique. Admittedly inadequate to the richness of human experience, these brief discussions may help the counselor to anticipate the emergence of major therapeutic issues and, with foreknowledge, to better manage the therapy.

These goals and themes are noted because they are the most common. That is not to say that for an individual any, or any combination, *must* emerge. Rarely is a theme purely articulated, without the intermingling of other themes. For instance, shame and guilt invariably also include family matters.

If none of these emerges, however, the absence is not unlike the dog that did not bark in the night. Gentle inquiries may be in order.

PSYCHOTHERAPEUTIC GOALS

Coming to Terms

One aspect of dealing with HIV chronic illness, with its rollercoaster and Sword of Damocles aspects, is in the goal of "coming to terms" with what is. By coming to terms, the client is not cured of HIV infection but is healed of his or her rage over an unjust world, and at fate that was determined by chance. With dissipation of rage often comes dissipation of depression, and the "acceptance" that Kübler-Ross (1969) noted. Wrote Kübler-Ross of the accepting client: "He will have been able to express his previous feelings, his envy for the living and the healthy, his anger at those who do not have to face their end so soon. He will have mourned the impending loss of so many meaningful people and places" (p. 112).

With this acceptance comes rejection of unhealthy grandiosity, a working through of anger, and a realization that the random, crazy world cannot answer such questions as "Why me?" The unjust world is forgiven, and with it many of those who have treated the client unjustly. The result can mean a freedom from the constrictions of emotional and physical insult, and a renewed ability to continue to live within the constrictions, discomforts, and fears. Kübler-Ross (1969) described this period as one that is not happy but, rather, void of feelings. However, this seems to be true only if the client is near death. The client who is able to come to terms sooner may not be "happy" exactly, but rather is at peace and satisfied with the realization that life continues and can be full of graces, but that it is different from the old life.

Is acceptance also the end of a fighting spirit? Should a therapist discourage a fighting spirit and encourage coming to terms? A reading of Kübler-Ross suggests that a fighting spirit is indicative of continuing denial, and that continuing to "struggle" precludes a death with peace and dignity—an interpretation which seems to include a value judgment requiring comment. For some, a death with dignity may require a fighting spirit to the end. Yet, who are we to take that away? It is unclear whether coming to terms with reality precludes hope or if acceptance suggests passivity. Perhaps what clients, and therapists, actually experience are complicated admixtures of acceptance and hope.

Connection and Reconnection

HIV clients are not like other clients. Some feel they historically have been excluded from society, in many different and personal ways. Some may have been rejected by family; many gay men will speak of how their fathers, reacting to their sons' "softness," distanced themselves. Persons with a history of drug use may never have felt part of society; some may be family "black sheep" or scapegoats. And those infected by heterosexual intercourse or transfusion may desperately hurt and feel separated from society. Many participate in their own exclusion by maintaining feelings of guilt, shame, and separateness. To achieve goals of connection and reconnection, the therapist acts as the agent who enables the client with a sociopolitically-loaded chronic illness to rejoin the family that is society.

The therapeutic goals for these clients may include self-acceptance, perhaps indicated by a new willingness to rejoin and feel a part of a community that will embrace them for the rest of their lives. In this, the therapist represents mother and father, neighborhood and society—the embodiment of a community that validates and appreciates the individual. It is the therapist's accepting stance that permits the new connection.

Planning for the Future

With AIDS now perceived as a chronic illness and the client's realization that life continues, therapy may deal with the question, "What do you want to do with the rest of your life?" That "rest of life" may stretch over a few months or many years. The period is, largely, unknown. This work within the context of an unpredictable chronic illness may include such concrete cognitive techniques as paper-and-pencil goal-setting, with time lines, or can include psychodynamic investigations of what has undermined goal attainment in the past. Nevertheless, this provides not only the therapist's communication of the importance of the client's future, but offers concrete criteria against which progress can be measured.

Other Therapy Goals

Other therapy goals to be considered may include:

- Education regarding the medical aspects of the illness, prevention, accommodation, and a healthy lifestyle.
- For those clients who seek an insight-oriented therapy, understanding of the dynamics of the past, with the goals of greater emotional well-being, new understandings with friends and caregivers, and greater courage.
- Exploration and resolution, or acceptance of nonresolution, of family issues.
- Exploration of issues of compliance and noncompliance with medical regimens.
- Preparation for death. This may take many forms, including acceptance and rapprochement, or may be more concrete, including the planning and drafting of wills, the consideration of do-not-resuscitate (DNR) orders, powers of attorney, and funeral planning.

PSYCHOTHERAPY THEMES

Therapy goals are not unrelated to psychotherapy themes. These are among the common themes expressed by HIV-positive persons:

Why Me?

The process of coming to terms is often begun with the client's question, "Why me?" With this question, two psychotherapeutic issues arise. The first is the emotional. In this regard, the client is not asking a question and knows there is no answer. Rather, anger and frustration are being expressed. When this occurs, follow the advice of my graduate school mentor, Wallace A. Kennedy, PhD, who often said, "Never interrupt a cry of agony." Listening to the emotion that underpins this question is what is needed here.

The second issue implied in the question is the social/political/theological theme of why tragic events occur and, more personally, why was the client the victim. Dostoyevski attempted to grapple with this question when one of the brothers Karamazov asked why God would allow a child to suffer. The Jews faced this issue in the Holocaust. Rabbi Harold Kushner (1981) provided some responses in his *When Bad Things Happen to Good People.* Many psychotherapists take an existential stance: that the world is an arena of many random, senseless, inexplicable occurrences, and AIDS is one of these. With this virus there have been many rolls of the dice. The HIV-positive client is now involved with a tragic epidemic in this century, and must be counseled with wisdom to find his or her own explanation that is based in wisdom rather than in angry blaming.

It's Not Me: Denial

The issue of denial is a complicated one and yet seems to lend itself to the most facile and glib of therapists' statements, the ubiquitous "the client's in denial." In fact, what appears to be "denial" can be understood and interpreted only by hearing the client's story. Without understanding the client's view of behaviors that may appear to be denial, one may make the premature assessment that a person who seems indifferent to the realities of HIV infection "is in denial." Rather, the contrary may be true: The person may already have grappled emotionally with HIV, decided it should not appreciably affect daily life, and is now living with appropriate but not undue concern.

Those who attempt to rush through the Kübler-Ross (1969) five stages make denial their primary target, and in doing so perform a grave disservice to the client. A client is not to be stripped unceremoniously of denial. Rather, the client, given a warm and secure therapeutic relationship, may then strip off the layers of denial, as they are no longer needed. If the client decides some layers of protection are still needed, only the arrogant clinician would have the audacity to strip the person bare.

The usual exception is that denial should be confronted when it interferes with a person's medical treatment. In the hospital setting, perceived denial that interferes with procedures is always confronted, and not always gently. However, a psychotherapist should be cautious when attributing the reluctance or refusal to seek treatment to denial; exploration may reveal other factors, including inappropriate hopelessness, cognitive impairment, psychosis, or a poor relationship with health care providers. Further, a client may decide he or she must make positive self-statements that are not actually believed but sound like denial. For example, a medical patient said to her doctor, "The virus will be out of my body in a month," and meant it as a statement of hope. A psychotherapist who understands the necessity of exploring "denial" will be less apt to make facile comments and is more likely to help the client find a proper balance of acceptance and hope.

Shame and Guilt

It has been suggested that guilt is felt for behaviors, while shame is felt for being a certain way or for belonging to a certain group. A guilt response is, "Look what I've done" while a shame response is "Look what a horrible person I am." Writers have suggested that shame is a painful experience, in which the client feels more like hiding than capable of repairing; guilt suggests some desire to make amends or repairs (Tangney, 1988; also Lewis, 1971; Lindsay-Hartz, 1984). With HIV-positive persons, psychotherapy is often spent on these emotions.

Persons with any of the risk factors—unsafe sex, heterosexual transmission, and intravenous drug use—may voice shame and guilt, albeit for different reasons. In gay men, HIV infection may underline and exacerbate historic guilt about homosexuality. IVDUs express guilt about having failed to accomplish much in life. Women, especially those infected heterosexually, feel guilty about their relationship with drug users or bisexuals.

Jeff, a 27-year-old Midwesterner, talked long about his parents and his anger about always having been made to feel ashamed of his femininity. Even as he laid in a hospital bed being treated for PCP, he was startlingly angry: "It was clear that my father started shunning me, maybe when I was 4 or 5. My brothers, they were more macho and he'd spend his time with them."

In another case, even as a gay man continued to live with AIDS, his parents suggested a girl friend, saying that she might help him with his illness, also implying (what was perhaps more important to them) that he could thereby improve his status in their eyes.

Some may handle the shame and guilt with facades. Ralph, a 35-year-old former high school teacher, admitted he created his artful facade because he believed his real self was too shameful. Among his artifices was one, and only one, very expensive made-to-measure suit. He'd wear it every Saturday night as he toured expensive New York bars, where he would play raconteur. He accepted free drinks from those who enjoyed his company, but that was always the extent of any relationships, because he believed if they knew him better, they would suspect his sordid secrets. The facade could never be threatened.

Ralph entered therapy because he was becoming depressed as HIV threatened his facade. He quickly saw the irony: KS lesions started to mark, and then spread over his face. Nevertheless, he gamely used makeup and continued his bar-hopping. Only in his final hospitalization was he able to set aside a bit of the facade, and then only a small piece. Perhaps it was the experience as a hospital patient, where little physical can be hidden, or perhaps his urgent physical situation suggested that there was little time left for pretenses.

Intravenous drug users, especially former users, discuss shame and guilt in terms of lost opportunities, and opportunities they never had. Their shame is not sexual, as it is with gays. Rather for some it emanates from the life of the street, where crimes, including selling oneself, to obtain drugs are shameful only when one is not high.

Women who contracted the virus through heterosexual intercourse often express guilt in terms of their failure, due to the illness, to care for dependents. Dependents are usually children, but sometimes are elderly parents. Many will excoriate themselves for not having been more careful in choice of sexual mate. Many of these women are the survivors—the male partner has already died. As such they bear the burden of continuing the family, and the guilt for failing to do so.

If the therapist begins to feel that the client is expressing inadequate guilt— that the client *should feel* guilt or even feel guiltier—then the practitioner's feelings should be explored in supervision. The therapist may be judging the client, placing blame, or in some way requiring penitence.

Abandonment

Genevieve had not walked for two months, and was being fed through a tube that led into a central vein. She had been cared for in a Bronx hospital, and then transferred to a nursing home which she left because of intense loneliness. Her three children were emotionally withdrawing from her, she said with sadness. She believed the departure was abetted by a social worker who had brought the children together to say goodbye to their mother. And yet, daily, she spoke of those children and her yearning to be home with them, and to have them play on her bed while she stroked their heads. She held on to them in her heart, even while she becoming increasingly debilitated and blind, due to CMV retinitis.

In our work with HIV-positive persons, indeed with most persons, one inescapable theme is that of separation and death. Death, as many philosophers have expressed, is at the heart of the existential anxiety that underlies much of this therapeutic work. Yalom's (1980) *Existential Psychotherapy,* full of anecdotes from his work with cancer patients, well describes existential issues and should be read by every practitioner in the HIV area.

Immediately and palpably, the existential anxiety of our clients is expressed in any number of ways. One patient suffered an anxiety attack when he was asked to enter the tube of the Magnetic Resonance Imaging (MRI) equipment. In therapy, he explained the unit reminded him of a coffin. Others express their existential anxiety as fear of loss of closeness. Many clients talk heartbreakingly of how they believe they will never be able to be held again, how they will never be able to make love again.

The loss of others is likely to have already occurred. Most HIV-positive persons are members of communities with others who preceded the client in illness and death. These losses are experienced as abandonments. As the client continues to live, more losses are always imminent. Martin (1988) has documented the emotionally eroding effects of repeated bereavements on gay men. Some persons who are HIV-positive through heterosexual intercourse or transfusions may feel abandoned because they suffer the stigma and the physical effects of the illness alone, without understanding. Others, such as a gay man who cared for his lover through illnesses and an AIDS-related death, may now be angry that no loving man will now care for him. Abandonment issues sometimes arise from a hospitalization, during which the muffled business of a death down the corridor is witnessed. In hospitals where PWAs are placed in the same units, these deaths are more often witnessed. If the therapist is aware of such an occurrence, he or she may want to raise the issue of the client's response to the death.

Abandonment fears also arise when the physical stigmata of the illness—weight loss or visible KS—are more apparent. In the therapy and in other relationships, the client may think or ask the question, "How can you stand to look at me?"; this may express self-disgust along with the fear that others will be disgusted and will abandon him or her.

If the therapist is willing to invite caregivers and friends to the sessions, this may be the forum for the client to discuss these concerns. The client should be cautioned beforehand that fantasized reassurances and renewed commitments may not necessarily result. What should result, guided by the therapist, is a more realistic view of the emotional capabilities of the caregivers and friends.

When abandonment does occur, one psychotherapeutic strategy is to help the client understand and, eventually, to forgive those who left. One patient said, plaintively, "My friends don't call me anymore. I mean, they know they can't catch the virus over the phone, but still they don't call." This client attributed the abandonment to his friends' fears of being infected. He was willing to consider, however, the possibility that these persons abandoned him now rather than be abandoned by him when he died.

For the therapist, too, abandonment may be a very difficult issue. For the therapist who sees down the road, the patient is a real presence who is here today but, due to the unpredictability of the illness, may not be present tomorrow. Ultimately, the client will not be physically present. To deal effectively with the client's feelings of abandonment, the therapist must have dealt with his or her past losses, or risk having those ghosts interfere in the therapeutic relationship, subtly or not. The therapist should not underestimate the difficulty in making a therapeutic commitment to someone who has a life-threatening illness. Indeed, it may seem soothing to say that this therapeutic relationship is analogous to all commitments we make: with lovers, spouses, parents, or children. None may be here tomorrow. But of course we do not think of *that;* our fear of their imminent loss is tucked away. Professional loss of the person with AIDS—be it in appointment cancellations, hospitalizations, or therapy breaks—portend the death and such losses are less easily ignored. If we feel subtle hints of sorrow during those temporary abandonments, imagine the anticipatory grief of the individual to whom loss is not theoretical, but imminently real.

Betrayal

One difficult issue for many is the sense that they were betrayed. One Hispanic man, in his last week of life, railed against the person who he believed infected him. "He knew," he said, "and yet he reassured me otherwise." Another man, discarding the clothes of a deceased lover, found evidence of infidelity, and cried bitterly during therapy. The work with betrayal is analogous to work with other losses. In this case, there is a loss of trust, or of a belief, that must be mourned.

Loss of Control and Dependency

Many were raised since potty training days to believe that being in control was, somehow, the *sine qua non* of existence. Along the way, despite occasional losses of control, we never became accustomed to not being totally in charge, with results totally within our grasp. Equally restricting were prohibitions against feeling or, especially, acting dependent. Better to drown than call for help, it seemed. Men especially were to be in control and independent, urged to stand up straight while hurting, and certainly not to cry. The women's movement advocated independence, but some interpreted that as a denial of natural dependent feelings in both men and women. If anything, we became ambivalent (ambivalence, it seems, is more acceptable) about control and dependency. Illness, especially serious acute and chronic illnesses, pulls us up short, and we are confronted with our lack of control and our dependencies.

Early on, HIV-positive persons become dependent on their prophylactic medication. As HIV infection progresses, other issues of dependency arise—involving medication, physicians, psychotherapists, friends, even canes.

With these issues, behaviors speak more eloquently than do words, especially in those not accustomed to psychotherapy. Behavior at one extreme is that of the patient who gives up all control and prefers to be cared for by physicians and other medical staff. This regression is more likely to be noticed by the psychotherapist who is approached by this client for additional attention. Often, the client does not discuss feelings about control, but talks about feelings of anger that he or she does not get additional time from medical personnel and, eventually, from the counselor.

At the other extreme is the patient who effectively walls himself or herself off from the outside world, fighting mightily against the feelings of dependence which are under the surface. Psychodynamic psychotherapists may see this as reaction formation. This client, in extreme manifestation, may not have a telephone or may seldom answer the telephone or make calls. This client may be sufficiently intelligent to know when medical treatment is necessary, but will delay seeking treatment. He or she is referred for noncompliance, but cannot understand the need to see a psychotherapist. Or, the person may be expressing some unhappiness, but not be able to account for the feelings.

Timing of interventions may be more crucial with this group than with others. Michael, a former advertising executive, was referred for therapy during a hospitalization for severe KS, which was then being treated with radiotherapy and alpha interferon. Said Michael, "I'm alone 95% of the time and basically like it that way. The other 5% of the time I'm with a nurse or social worker or someone like you, and I tolerate it." He described his relationship with his mother as intellectually stimulating but devoid of emotional communication. He had no phone in his hospital room, and no visitors. He spent much of his time watching television and reading: escaping intellectually. Despite that, he was aware that his illness was serious, and he could no longer dam up his yearnings for closeness. The time had come for soul-searching, he realized. During the second session, Michael said he had some distant friends he would like to speak with. The first therapy goal was his obtaining a phone. After the phone was installed, the goal of calling them was agreed upon. It took another week, but he made the calls. He died two weeks later.

Quick recognition of dependency issues, and how the client plays them out, may prevent early termination. The help-seeker may become frustrated and apprehensive with the therapist who too early suggests less dependency. The help-rejector may be intrigued by an early, gentle interpretation of the walled-off stance. Reframing is useful. For nursing and medical staff, a gentle response to a help-rejector is this simple statement: "I know it makes you uncomfortable when I do certain things for you. But it's my job to take care of you in some ways. Please just let me do my job."

Fear of Dying

Randall was a 40-year-old man who looked 25 years old: a man with a quick smile and an apparent carefree nature who was far from carefree. Always anxious, with a textbook case of panic disorder, he was more ruminative than usual one Friday. A hospital employee had inadvertently left his chart open, and he saw his latest CD-4 cell count before his internist was able to gently provide those numbers. The count was 128. He had just memorialized his lover, who had died two years ago that month. He was thinking of his own dying.

"I'm not afraid of death. I pray every night. I go to Mass on Sundays, and I'm a believer that God will welcome me. But I'm still afraid of the dying process. It wasn't so great for my lover; I managed that time ok, but I don't want my family to go through my dying. I don't want them to see me curled up and wasting away. I don't want them coming in and seeing me with tubes in my arms and up my nose. It's dying that I'm concerned about."

Randall went on to say that he did not look forward to dying, but he insisted that his concern was for his family; they would be upset, not he.

With time, Randall would become a little less oblique about his dying fears, and he would "own" more of those feelings that he initially projected on his family.

Expression of these fears usually includes several related concerns: That the dying will be painful and labored, which can be addressed by the physician who can explain pain control; that it will be shameful, with loss of control of bodily function; that it will come after a long period of dementia (after "being a vegetable"), or that it will occur while alone, which may be realistic, depending on the social support system and hospital rules.

Along with the emotional exploration of these concerns, the therapist can also help the patient talk about how he or she would like the dying to be—in essence, to plan the dying and death. This discussion may include location (home or hospital), the persons the client would want nearby, what the client would want those persons to do (pray, sing, tell stories), and the memorial service. The discussion may also include what messages the client would like to leave behind, either by telling people before the death, or by writing or videotaping.

Loss of Future

Many persons with HIV infection perceive their lives as foreshortened. The increasing chronicity of the illness has little affected this perception. Anger and sadness due to loss of future is voiced by persons who have been successful in life, those who found successes only recently and others who admit they squandered their past and mourn the loss of a future that might have been. These hopes and dreams for the future may often include hopes for another generation and are typified by expressions regarding loss of ability to procreate, or inability to see children grow and prosper.

A former IVDU, referred initially for psychiatric treatment for atypical facial pain, had ceased drug use in 1983. He went through a drug-free program, began to work for a large corporation in an accounting position, and was raising an adolescent daughter. With his third AIDS hospitalization came discussion that his future was stolen from him. "I got myself going. I gave myself a life. I stopped using drugs. But it [HIV] came back from my past and got me now."

As with others confronting potential loss, clients have remarkable responses: new intensity regarding life and relationships and new commitments to unfulfilled tasks, among them. The practitioner may want to observe that emotionally charged behaviors may be the client's way to affirm life. One client told how he and his lover spent the weekend in very dramatic arguments, with much yelling, crying, and screaming. It seemed that an emotionally intense argument was his way of reasserting life, even as he mourned the loss of his future.

A Life of Unknowing

One of the most common themes voiced by HIV-positive persons is the "not knowing" about the course the illness will take, including when a crisis will arise. It is often put in terms of an erosive, stressful lifestyle, with continual taking of medications serving as reminders several times a day, and with no opportunity to escape from either the condition or the reminders. Said one person, angrily describing day-to-day life, "I have to take medicine every four hours, but even then I'm not sure if it's worth it. I get an ache, I worry that it's another AIDS problem. When I can't sleep, I worry. What I need is a vacation from this illness."

Some professionals report anecdotally that persons with ARC seem the most anxious of HIV-positive persons, because their symptoms are somewhat vague and not serious enough for an AIDS diagnosis. That anxiety decreases with an AIDS diagnosis, some say, because the other shoe has dropped and the course of illness is perceived to be clearer.

While the actual AIDS diagnosis may at one level be a relief, at another it is a source for anxiety based on the considerable vicissitudes of the illness, which are not knowable and which can be controlled only somewhat.

The client may ask some variation of the question, "Because I can't be cured, wouldn't it be better to give up?" This question often expresses a great weariness and the question within may be, "Is my life worth living despite the discomfort and pain?" The question may also serve to ask the psychotherapist for some affirmation of the importance and value of life, especially in the face of AIDS. More particularly, the client may be asking the therapist for a statement regarding the value of the client.

Living Fully

"Courage is self-affirmation 'in spite of,' that is in spite of that which tends to prevent the self from affirming itself," wrote Tillich in *The Courage to Be* (1952, p. 32).

The task for us all, including the HIV-positive person, is to live life fully "in spite of." In spite of handicaps, infirmities, an uncertain course, and, certainly, death. The HIV-positive person doubtless carries heavy burdens, made heavier by anxiety based in the fear of death. But fear can be met with courage, Tillich reminds us.

The psychotherapist's task is help the client name and face the fear, thereby finding the courage to live more fully. To different persons, this will mean different things. A mother may want to spend more time with a daughter. A writer may want to finish a play. Another may just want to be able to work a few more months. Others may want to speak unsaid things, make phone calls that should have been made years ago.

Family Issues

Those who present with family issues have few complaints that are not longstanding. These may include feelings of unacceptability, with the source in the family. Some gay men may report early rejection by the father, and those with an IVDU history may report growing up in a dysfunctional family, or being scapegoated and shunned by relatives. Family members may express anger at the son's, daughter's, or siblings' unacceptable, even "perverted," behaviors.

One gay man, Robert, talked in sessions about his yearnings to have a relationship with his father. Childhood memories he recalled included his father taking canoe trips with a sibling, while Robert stayed at home. The early perceived loss of the father as a caring figure is generally expressed as a sorrowful continued yearning, but rarely is there optimism about reconciliation. The client continues to perceive the father as rejecting and ungiving. Jeff, who remained without hope of conciliation, would talk to his mother by phone daily, but his father never came to the phone.

The client generally refuses to see any possibility of reconciliation and adamantly believes there can be none. Parents and siblings, too, may be unable to set aside deeply felt prejudices, and may justify them on religious and cultural grounds. The therapist may find himself or herself in the middle: Relatives may view the clinician as an ally of perversion, and the client may distort the clinician into a parental figure, with consequent anger and yearning.

Rapprochement of disaffected family members is often a fantasy of the therapist, which should be faced in supervision and not foisted on the client. The client will perceive this accurately as the therapist's wish, as pressure misguided in the face of impossibility, and (familiar) pressure to conformity. The idea of rapprochement certainly has occurred to the client. It is important here to discern accurately the therapy theme: Is it the possibility of reconciliation, or is it the yearning for or anger about a reconciliation that can never occur? To mistake one for the other may indicate the therapist's feelings are inappropriately involved here.

Another family issue may be the client's having to deal with parents' continuing unrealistic expectations for their adult child. One family told their adult son, who to their shame had long lived a gay lifestyle, that if he only found a woman the AIDS situation would be resolved.

Another effect of HIV is that generational succession has been turned on its head. Normally, adult children are expected to care for and bury their parents. With AIDS, many elderly parents are caring for and burying their adult children. The client may feel responsibility for the parents, and feel that they will be abandoned both economically and emotionally during the chronic illness and after his or her death. The adult child may fear as much for the parent's well-being, after the death from AIDS, as for his or her own well-being. This may result in misguided attempts to save money by avoiding needed medical care, or in added guilt that exacerbates longstanding feelings.

Financial Concerns

Among all patients, rich and poor, there is concern regarding subsistence for themselves and for others in their family systems. Intermingled are issues of pride, dependency, and feeling productive and useful. As mentioned in Chapter 3, patients face hard decisions about paying many thousands of dollars annually in uninsured medical costs versus going on public assistance. The assistance may help financially but is psychologically corrosive. Others mourn the loss of their assets—really, what they represent in terms of achievement and comforts—to pay medical bills. Often, clients may use psychotherapy to help their decision-making, regarding such issues as going on public assistance, selling property, accepting the financial help of family and friends, and leaving work.

Envy of the Healthy

A man with fresh-faced looks laid back in his bed and said, "I almost hate to have visitors. I mean, I'm 29 and maybe I shouldn't feel this way, but I look at them and they're healthy and they're living their lives. I'm envious." This envy may extend to the psychotherapist, who is perceived as healthy, as well as to visitors.

Relationships with Medical Professionals

I've been asking the doctor when I'll get to go home. She keeps saying maybe in two weeks.
When she says maybe, what do you hear?
I hear "no," that I won't go home.

Good communications between the HIV-positive patient and medical professionals can be problematic, oftentimes due to the emotional charge of the illness for both parties. Other reasons for communication problems may include dementia, which creates forgetfulness, or class or cultural differences. It should be remembered that poor communications are seldom the fault of one party, but usually the result of the interaction of both parties.

With this matter, as with others, the therapist may have to move along the therapeutic continuum, ranging from problem solving to case-management function in which the therapist would discuss problems with the doctors, or give a client permission to change physicians. When those relationships become a therapy issue, the therapist's task initially should be to encourage and empower the client to improve those communications. Problem-solving techniques can include: Encouraging the client to write questions and concerns before the appointment and, in advance, asking the health care provider for additional time to discuss questions and concerns.

Disclosure

The client may be reticent to disclose his or her medical situation to family or friends. Often, the client will say the knowledge would hurt a weak member of the family. Upon some investigation, the therapist may discern that the person being protected is actually the client, because the disclosure would bring up issues that he or she has kept from the family. Shame and guilt may be involved, and, possibly, a lengthy history of hiding an alternative lifestyle. With disclosure of HIV infection, all the issues around the lifestyle will be revealed. Fears of abandonment or the client's anger regarding abandonment that has already occurred may also be explored. Another possible course of inquiry may be based on the psychodynamic defense of projection. The client may be projecting fears and unease on family members.

It is also important to explore whether the client is failing to acknowledge love and support that may actually exist. A mother seeking psychotherapy expressed great anger because a son and daughter colluded in keeping his AIDS secret. When she found out, she had only 2 months left with her son before he died. She was angry: "They cheated me out of more time with my son. I could've spent more time with him, enjoyed him more, been with him more. But they cut me out of the picture."

This listing of themes is hardly exhaustive, but rather serves as a device to help the psychotherapist anticipate what may arise in sessions with an HIV-positive person. Each person, of course, will provide very personal expressions of these themes, and is likely to add many others.

6
Therapist's Monitoring Function

The PWA, a former intravenous drug user, was blind from CMV-related retinitis. He spent several weeks in the hospital, and then returned home, to be cared for by family members and a home health attendant. The family maintained almost daily contact with the hospital staff physician who cared for the patient. They asked him questions about the blindness, about his eating and sleeping. But only when they brought the patient to the emergency room was it discovered that the patient had gone 20 days without a bowel movement.

In another case, a woman with HIV infection was seen by a therapist who noted that the client seemed to have difficulty maintaining arousal and paying attention. The client, usually crisply alert, was babbling. The person "didn't seem to be the same."

The subspecialty of psychotherapy with HIV-infected persons differs from other clinical work because the therapist must not only be knowledgeable about the various related physical and psychiatric conditions, but must also act as monitor for emergent symptoms.

It is a task made more important because family members, friends, and other caregivers may fail to recognize and respond to physical and mental changes that can signal serious complications. Some caregivers simply have inadequate knowledge or resources to recognize that a change in mentation, for example, may indicate a serious physical problem. Others fail to intervene based on their concepts of autonomy or out of their own denial or hopes for improvements. Hope and denial are heard in such comments as, "We waited, hoping tomorrow it may disappear," and "I have an appointment with my doctor next week. It can wait."

Other explanations given for slow responses include perceived unavailability of medical consultation ("My doctor's too busy"), the community's emergency room situation ("Rather than sit there for eight hours, I'll hope it is just a passing phase"), transportation problems, and a reluctance to summon emergency help because of embarrassment and fear the neighbors will learn of one's condition. Whatever the actual psychodynamic, family-systems, or cognitive reasons, clients' and caregivers' failure to react quickly to an emergent crisis may merit any number of productive psychotherapy sessions.

The psychotherapist, however, must have the knowledge to recognize an out-of-the-ordinary situation—such as heightened anxiety, depression, and delirium—and the resolve to respond quickly, unencumbered by emotional issues. The signals of organic problems and the necessary responses are discussed in the first part of this chapter. Moreover, the therapist must expertly deal with a competent client's refusal to seek help or to comply with medical regimens, as well as with suicidal ideation and intent. These are discussed in the latter part of the chapter.

SYMPTOMS VERSUS CAUSES

HIV-related illnesses, clearly complicated, often present with psychiatric or mental-status symptoms which are puzzling, at least initially, even to physicians. Issues such as the physical and mental effects of drug use and withdrawal further complicate the picture. When a client is having puzzling symptoms, the psychotherapist should avoid making statements regarding the possible causes. Such statements, outside the practitioners' competence, may unduly alarm the client, create additional anxiety that may lead to increased inertia or despair, and may slow the client's help-seeking. Moreover, such efforts can create liabilities that would be difficult to defend before a state board or jury. The therapeutic response to the client who is evidencing troubling symptoms may be couched like this, "I noticed that you are breathing with a lot of difficulty after climbing my one flight of stairs. This hasn't happened before. Would you consider telephoning your physician before you leave my office and explain the problem, and that I am concerned. Then let's see what she says." If the client is reluctant to act, then that reluctance should be discussed. If there are clear symptoms of an emergency, the therapist must gauge the danger to the client and whether the client is being realistic about the situation. The clinician must be be willing to intervene despite the patient's wishes, if the danger is great or the client is unable to articulate a realistic understanding of the situation and the ramifications of failing to seek medical help.

INDICATORS OF MEDICAL EMERGENCY

In many cases, despite an emergent medical situation, social functioning remains intact and provides a deceptive "cover" of normality. Conversely, reluctance to seek help may be expressed vaguely or illogically, or the patient may be unable to express comprehension of the gravity of the situation. While not all symptoms of a medical emergency can be anticipated, the following are the most common signs of a major organic problem.

1. Difficulties in communicating.

- Aphasia: inability to speak.
- Dysphasia: difficulties speaking.

Difficulty speaking generally points to central nervous system involvement and requires immediate intervention. For example, one possible presenting symptom of cryptococcal meningitis is mutism.

2. Hallucinations.

- Visual.
- Auditory.
- Olfactory.

These too may indicate organic involvement and require prompt medical intervention. Visual hallucinations or vivid dreams can be side effects of antituberculosis (anti-TB) regimens. Hallucinations also sometimes accompany high fevers or delirium.

3. Other acute cognitive impairment.

These can be tested by questions regarding orientation, and by memory and calculations tests, and other examinations (Berg, Franzen, & Wedding, 1987; Mueller, 1984). The assessment instruments should be sensitive to brain impairment. Sudden changes in cognition are distinct from the chronic picture of dementia, symptoms of which include subtle memory loss over time. If a person normally has relatively good memory and calculation skills and an acute impairment is evident, medical intervention is necessary.

4. Delirium.

The symptoms of delirium include rapid onset (acuteness); disorientation to time, place, or person; memory impairment; inability to maintain arousal or attention; disorganized thinking; and incoherent speech. (Consult the DSM-III-R [*Diagnostic and Statistical Manual of Mental Disorders,* 3rd. ed., *Revised*] American Psychiatric Association, 1987, p. 103.) Acute agitation in PWAs is often the result of delirium. The causes can be many, and should be left to the physician for diagnosis. Although psychiatric medications are sometimes used to calm the agitation, hospitalization is required both to protect the patient and to find the physical cause.

5. Significant shortness of breath or chest pain.

Either significant shortness of breath or chest pain may indicate respiratory problems. The client usually complains about these, but the therapist may notice the problem, and should discuss it. Ancillary complaints may include dizziness after brief exertion or great fatigue after brief exertion. Lack of oxygen may lead to anxiety that cannot be explained by the client.

6. Fever.

If an HIV-positive person is aware of a condition that causes fever, such as MAI, then careful attention should be paid to any increases in fever. If no cause of fever is known, then attention should be paid to chronic fever, especially if there are "spikes" or sudden increases.

7. Headaches.

Headaches seem part and parcel of life and have many etiologies. However, when a patient without prior history of headaches (tension or migraine, for example) complains of headaches, this merits a referral to the physician. Standard medical care, especially with HIV-positive persons, requires a diagnostic CAT (computer axial tomographic) scan for headaches of unknown origin.

8. Seizure activity.

Any indication of seizures requires immediate action.

9. Incontinence.

Incontinence of urine or feces requires prompt attention.

PSYCHIATRIC MANIFESTATIONS OF THE ILLNESS

The psychotherapist must also be alert to the possibility of psychiatric disorders, that is, those amenable to psychopharmacological as well as psychotherapeutic interventions. These may be preexisting conditions, such as bipolar disorder, or may be directly caused by HIV or occur in reaction to HIV. *Any psychiatric symptom may be a presentation of HIV infection* in an individual with risk behaviors or known HIV infection, and a referral to a competent clinician is required. A discussion of some psychiatric problems common to HIV-positive persons, and treatment, follows.

Depression and Anxiety

Mood disorders seem to comprise the majority of psychiatric manifestations to HIV infection. These may be preexisting, or in reaction to, or caused by HIV infection.

Baer (1989) detailed the diagnoses of 60 persons with AIDS or ARC treated on a locked inpatient unit. Despite the fact that (except for those with dementia) the causes of disorders could not be certainly ascribed to HIV, nevertheless 60% of these persons had their first psychiatric hospitalization since infection. The majority had mixtures of psychopathology, but the primary diagnosis of 20 was depression. Eighteen were diagnosed with at least moderate dementia, six had symptoms of schizophrenia (waiving the DSM-III-R stipulation requiring the ruling out of organic process), six had brief reactive psychoses, and four were diagnosed with manic bipolar disorder. The remainder had adjustment disorder or stimulant-related psychoses. For the adjustment disorders and brief reactive psychoses, stressors included the newly diagnosed disease, loss of a love relationship, housing and financial crises, and perception of progression of the illness.

Perry et al. (1990), using diagnostic instruments with persons seeking HIV testing, found rates of current mood disorders in all subjects and current alcohol and nonintravenous substance dependence higher than in a catchment area sample. Lifetime rates of mood disorders and nonalcohol substance abuse in all subjects was roughly double that in a catchment control sample.

In general, depressive symptoms may range from the adjustment disorder with depressed mood to major depression. The clinician should be warned, however, that the diagnostic criteria must be well scrutinized to avoid technical errors, but even then some catchall diagnoses may be required. DSM-III-R (APA, 1987) criteria for adjustment disorder include maladaptive reaction indicated either by impairment in social and occupational functioning or by symptoms in excess of a normal and expectable reaction. Further, the maladaptive reaction should last no more than 6 months. Adjustment disorder with depressed mood "should be used when the predominant manifestation is symptoms such as depressed mood, tearfulness, and feelings of hopelessness" (APA, 1987, p. 331). But what is the diagnosis for the chronically dysphoric HIV-positive person who maintains some semblance of occupational functioning? Perhaps the catchall, Adjustment Disorder Not Otherwise Specified, can be used.

For a formal diagnosis of major depressive episode, five symptoms are required, as well other criteria. However, among the list of criteria symptoms are many common physical complaints voiced by PWAs, including significant weight loss, daily fatigue or loss of energy, and sleep problems. If the criteria are taken literally, many PWAs will already have three to four symptoms by virtue of their physical situation. This problem is illustrated further by a Beck Depression Inventory (BDI; Beck, Ward, Mendelson, Mock, & Erbaugh, 1961, survey of hospitalized AIDS patients). Because the BDI has many questions regarding physical complaints, responses to these inflated the total BDI score, leading to indications of depression in patients reporting a nondepressed mood (Winiarski & Hoffman, 1990). Diagnosis and treatment of depression in HIV-positive and HIV-symptomatic persons should rely less on the physical manifestations and instead focus on the client's feelings and thoughts, including mood, feelings about death, guilt, and feelings of worthlessness and despair.

Many patients with adjustment disorders should respond to cognitive psychotherapy. Research indicates effectiveness of medicine and cognitive behavioral therapy (Miller, Norman, & Keitner, 1989). Ayd (1988) suggests only small doses of a benzodiazepine for concurrent anxiety and insomnia.

Patients with major depressions require psychiatric assessment for medication. To those reluctant to take antidepressants, I explain that the medication allows for additional "psychological space. . . . When some people are depressed, they can't marshal their resources to fight back. The antidepressant gives them more emotional space and strength to gather their resources."

Psychiatrists use a variety of antidepressants. Prozac (fluoxetine), neither a tricyclic nor an MAOI, is becoming more widely used due to patients' quick response, which usually occurs in days, and its activating effects. If the patient feels too activated, the daily dosage is reduced. One method of reducing the dose requires having the client empty the capsule into a liquid and drinking a fraction of that liquid. Other antidepressants used include Pamelor or Aventyl (nortriptyline), Norpramin (desipramine), or Desyrel (trazodone) started in low doses with gradual increments to a therapeutic dose. (Note that priapism has an incidence of 1 in 1000 to 10000 with trazodone.) Blood levels of nortriptyline or desipramine can be measured to help titrate the dose and check compliance. Sinequan (doxepin) generally is not recommended due to its anticholinergic effects.

Some HIV-positive patients who seem to have diminished mental abilities improve with stimulant therapy. Fernandez, Adams, et al. (1988) used methylphenidate (Ritalin) and dextroamphetamine to treat 10 ARC patients. Side effects were absent and improvements in cognitive functioning were noted in all but one subject. Notable but not statistically significant were the findings that frontal lobe dysfunction responded preferentially to methylphenidate while dysmnesias and affective symptomatology responded preferentially to dextroamphetamine. In clinical practice, dosages range from 5 to 15 mg taken several times a day, but no later than 4 P.M. (Ayd, 1985; see also Holmes, Fernandez, & Levy, 1989; Fernandez, Levy, & Galizz, 1988.)

Anxiety Disorders

The presentation of anxiety in an HIV-positive person illustrates the necessity of the psychotherapist's monitoring function and the importance of the clinician's willingness to convince the client to seek immediate help.

Any presentations of anxiety should set off warning signals for the therapist. A quick referral back to the client's physician and, if necessary, a visit to the emergency room may be indicated if several factors are present:

1. if the anxious feelings cannot be clearly attributed to a current psychological factor (such as, "I've been thinking about death a lot" or, "I am thinking about telling my parents"). Typically in this type of case, the client expresses surprise and concern about the symptoms and cannot explain why they are occurring.
2. when such symptoms are atypical for the client even when psychologically stressed.
3. if the symptoms are extreme; normal coping mechanisms are failing and the client feels the anxiety is out of control.
4. when physical symptoms are concurrent. These may include shortness of breath, however mild; headaches; or subtle seizure activity.

This careful monitoring is necessary because the differential diagnoses for anxiety in an HIV-positive person, or a person with risk factors but not proven HIV-negative, are many and complex. Causative factors can include but are not restricted to: hypoxia due to an incipient respiratory disorder; onset of a functional or organic psychosis; metabolic disorders; substance (including methadone) withdrawal, cocaine intoxication, or several simultaneous processes. (For medical causes of anxiety, see Rosenbaum & Pollack, 1987.)

When organic factors are ruled out by a physician, anxiety disorders can range—in the terminology of the diagnostic systems—from adjustment disorders with anxious mood to panic disorder, which may be associated with HIV-related concerns or may be the result of an exacerbation of a preexisting condition. One client, for example, suffered panic attacks when asked to enter the tube of a CAT scanner.

A nonpharmacological and efficacious psychological treatment for anxiety is stress innoculation (Meichenbaum, 1985). This cognitive-behavioral treatment allows the client to choose from a "menu" of techniques to reduce stress. These skills, taught to the client, include relaxation training, cognitive strategies, and problem-solving strategies. (See also Barlow, 1988, for explication of treatments for anxiety.)

Ayd (1988) suggests a low dose of Ativan (lorazepam) or Xanax (alprazolam) with a short course to avoid benzodiazepine dependency. For insomnia, some psychiatrists in AIDS settings prefer Restoril (temazepam) to Halcion (triazolam) because Halcion's short half life causes some patients to awake in the middle of the night (Salzman, 1990).

Mania

One psychiatric manifestation of HIV infection is mania in persons with no previous history of such disorder. While the dangers of a manic episode are well known, these may be compounded if an HIV-infected person's symptoms include additional sexual activities. If the manic patient is hospitalized, Ayd (1988) suggests use of intravenous haloperidol (Haldol) to quell an acute attack, with Symmetrel (amantadine) if an extrapyramidal reaction occurs. Longterm treatment generally employs lithium carbonate. This medication, which can be toxic in too-high doses and damaging to kidney and thyroid, requires careful patient management including regular blood level monitoring.

Following a report that lithium may improve patients' white blood counts (which are depressed by zidovudine and other HIV-fighting drugs), some doctors prescribe lithium to leukopenic patients. This use, too, requires careful monitoring with frequent blood levels taken. In one case, a patient transferred from another hospital reported gait problems and some confusion, which was quickly diagnosed by a neurologist as lithium overdose. Note also that a report also links hypomania with use of Elavil (amitriptyline) (Holmes & Fricchione, 1989).

Delirium

Agitation that accompanies delirium is symptomatically treated by Haldol (haloperidol) which can also cause delirium and should be discontinued if the condition worsens (Ayd, 1988). Philip Muskin, MD, associate chief of the consultation-liaison service at Presbyterian Hospital, New York, recommends a 100 mg dose of Thorazine (chlorpromazine) to control acute agitation. These treatments are intended to serve as behavioral management aids, while physicians search for the physical causes of the condition (personal communication, May, June, 1989).

Baer (1989) cautioned that demented patients in his study "evidenced considerable intolerance of haloperidol" (p. 1287), with two cases of urinary retention and six cases of severe extrapyramidal reactions, although these patients were taking antiparkinsonian medication. For extrapyramidal reactions—indicated by neck twisting, for example—Symmetrel (amantadine) is recommended because of its low anticholinergic effects.

DELIBERATE REFUSAL TO SEEK TREATMENT

Oftentimes, for various reasons, a client will refuse to seek medical attention. This *requires* a thorough exploration, with an assessment of the appropriateness of the client's response.

A competent client has the right to refuse treatment; however, this ideally falls within the context of a thoroughly explored philosophy, with clear understanding of benefits and risks. If despair and hopelessness are involved in a refusal to seek treatment, or if the decision is spontaneous and not consistent with a previously articulated stance, the therapist must assess the appropriateness of the thinking. Factors to consider include:

- Is the emotional content proportionate to the situation? Refusal to seek treatment may be rationally justified by a person who is in the end stages of illness and who wants to avoid further medical procedures. This situation contrasts significantly with that of treatment-refusal by a person experiencing the first PCP-related hospitalization, and with a positive prognosis.
- If a person with AIDS is refusing treatment, is the reaction due to lack of knowledge regarding HIV illness generally, or to the current situation specifically? Does the patient trust and understand his physician's prognostic statements?
- Is distrust, even paranoia, or a preexisting oppositional stance involved?
- Is the client catastrophizing, with thinking influenced by a preexisting depression? A psychiatric disorder may be interactive, including heightened anxiety which the patient believes will be relieved by death, or clinical depression. HIV-related organic mental syndrome, which can cloud thinking, may also be contributory.

Related are the issues of "living wills" and "do-not-resuscitate orders." A Living Will, such as the one suggested by the National Council on Death and Dying (see Appendix), can be a detailed listing of what medical interventions an individual may or may not wish in a medical emergency. The document has different force in different jurisdictions. A DNR order may be requested by a physician from a patient or the person who holds the patient's medical power of attorney. Depending on the governmental, community, and hospital norms, these orders are more or less detailed, asking the patient to consider interventions which can be maintained or not used. While some hospitals may ask patients to consider DNR orders as a matter of course, most wait until a patient is seriously ill.

Much discussion of these has been made, but without stressing the possibility that these documents may be appropriate at some times, and in some situations in a person's life, but not in others. A healthy man in his 30s is very likely to want cardiopulmonary resuscitation if he stops breathing after an automobile accident; an 80-year-old with cancer may not want such heroic methods if she stops breathing in a hospital bed.

Only one correct stance exists on these issues: The necessity of the therapist's conscious neutrality while discussing issues of life and death with the client. Competent practice requires nothing less than the therapist having already considered his or her personal stance on the right to die and attempting to prevent, if necessary with great effort, that personal stance from influencing the psychotherapy.

SUICIDE

Suicidal ideation is very common with HIV-infected persons. The meager research available and anecdotal reports (Frierson & Lippmann, 1988, for example) indicate there is significant suicide risk.

Holland and Tross (1985), early in the AIDS epidemic, stated that suicides were actually uncommon among PWAs. Years later, others are not so sure. Marzuk et al. (1988) studied suicides in New York City in 1985 and calculated the suicide rate among male AIDS patients between ages 20 to 59 was 66.15 times that of the general population and 36.3 times that of men without AIDS in the same age group. These findings were based on 12 suicides of men ages 20 to 59 who were known to have AIDS. Eight were homosexual or bisexual; the risk factor of four were unknown. Other than the possibility of IVDUs being among the four "unknowns," no drug users were included in these statistics. In response, Kizer, Green, Perkins, Doebbert, & Hughes (1988) noted their data indicate "the relative risk of suicide for California men with AIDS was 17.02 times that of men without AIDS" (p. 1881). Others critized Marzuk et al.'s methodologies (Beltangady, 1988; Hull, Sewell, Wilson, & McFeeley, 1988). Other authors (Frierson & Lippmann, 1988) describe case reports. Data from general hospitals, not involving AIDS patients, led Goldberg (1987) to suggest that a hospital will experience about one suicide per 20,000 admissions.

Many philosophic issues become involved when suicide is mentioned. Some believe no suicide can be rational, that is, well thought-out and not caused by a psychiatric condition. Others will argue for a person's right to have a well thought-out "rational" suicide, especially in the face of debilitating illness. Others note that self-neglect may be suicidal, citing Schneidman (1983), who suggests that subintentional suicide may be acted out in seemingly unrelated self-destructive acts.

Other issues whose study can be important in clinical applications include: Can we identify a subset of PWAs, such as drug users, who are more likely to attempt suicide? Should strict limits be put on take-home medications for those persons? Should we treat every drug overdose as a suicide attempt? If a person with a good prognosis declines life-extending medical aid, is this a manifestation of suicidal behavior requiring intervention?

The clinician who works with HIV-infected persons realizes quickly that suicidal ideation is commonplace and often a topic for discussion. Discussion of such ideation should provoke inquiry, rather than panic. A routine but gentle assessment should be made with, as described by Goldberg (1987), a series of nonthreatening questions that escalate to specificity. He suggested, for instance, that an initial question may be related to the possibility of discouragement, followed by "I wonder if there are times when you think about your situation and it makes you feel like crying?" (p. 447). The next question he suggested is, "Did you ever feel that if your life were to go on like this that it just wouldn't be worth living?" (p. 447). Questions about a plan and means would follow, if appropriate. Many will say they have thought about suicide but are not suicidal. Others have fantasized not an active suicide but rather "going to sleep" or "being put out of my misery." Those who speak about suicide should asked about:

1. Imminence: Many persons say they are not immediately suicidal but think about it in case they were to become extremely debilitated.
2. Provocation: Has something occurred that makes the client think about suicide now? Does the person feel a certain way now?
3. Plan, including the method: Does the patient have a well thought-out plan, or is it a vague notion?
4. Means: Does the patient have at his or her disposal the means to suicide? Many PWAs have been prescribed many pills, and hoarding those pills may be indicative of intent.

An important consideration for the practitioner is an assessment of presence of delirium. If there is any clouding of consciousness, changes in awareness, or perceptual disturbances, the client may not be a reliable informant or may not be able to inhibit dangerous impulses (Goldberg, 1987). The therapist's decision regarding actual danger is a judgment call, but one that should be made with a backup—a colleague psychiatrist who can begin hospitalization.

Discussions of suicide are often cries for help. It is commonly known that a psychotherapist would have to block such an attempt. It is likely, then, that the patient who raises serious discussion of suicide believes the therapist will either collude in the plan or block it.

Psychotherapists, depending on training and their own feelings, have varied responses to threats of suicide. One person told her Roman Catholic patient, "It's a mortal sin." The effectiveness of that tactic is unclear. Another counselor works out of an Eastern-oriented view in which the problems of this life are not evaded by suicide, but return in the next life to be worked out there. A well-thought-out stance on suicide is very important in helping the practitioner to maintain equilibrium in the face of a threat that can provoke extreme anxiety. If there is a clear danger, the therapist has a professional responsibility to intervene in a fashion that does not exacerbate the client's emotional state. But what if the practitioner agrees with the client's decision? What if the danger is unclear, such as in cases of withdrawing from treatment? The practitioner should consider these cases now, and attempt to understand his or her feelings regarding them, before such a case is presented in a session.

Anticipatory Agreement Regarding Intervention

Well-trained psychotherapists know that they have the professional responsibility to intervene decisively if a client's life is in danger, or if the client endangers others. As of this writing, there are no known major cases involving the issues of therapist's or medical manager's breach of confidentiality in order to intervene when an emergency is suspected. Goldberg (1987), writing about suicide, suggested asking a third party about the client's suicidal ideation. If the client, however, does not give permission, then the practitioner must make the decision "based on prevailing attitudes towards the rights of patients. Generally, clinicians can override the refusal of a patient in this area if they deem the situation to be of some potential and immediate life-threatening nature" (Goldberg, 1987, p. 450). In small towns, where AIDS stigma may persist, the breach of confidentiality may seem more severe. In larger cities with more PWAs, the resulting stigma may be less severe. Nevertheless, the medical issues of HIV infection are very complicated, and may require the therapist to take professional risks to protect the patient's physical well-being.

One possible solution to such dilemmas is an anticipatory agreement made with the client in the early stages of psychotherapy. The therapist may broach the subject, at the appropriate time, saying, "I understand your concern about the physical aspects of AIDS. And I know you know that sometimes a person may suddenly become ill, and then may not realize how serious the situation is. If I see something like that, how would you want me to handle it?" The patient normally will appreciate the caring.

Sometimes an agreement anticipating a specific concern may be appropriate. In one case, I made an agreement with a patient who had dementia, lived alone, and had no social support system: If you miss a session and I do not hear from you within 8 hours, I will call the police to check your apartment.

Without these types of anticipatory agreements, decisive action may have to be taken. A 55-year-old Hispanic man, who showed signs of dementia, telephoned his therapist in mid-October and explained that he could not make his September 23 appointment. He said his feet were too swollen and he could not walk. Additional inquiry indicated the client was not oriented to time. The clinician urged him to go to the emergency room. When he demurred, the therapist decided that the patient's mental status required decisive intervention. The client was told to be in the ER in two hours, or emergency medical services would be summoned. The therapist then also contacted the client's physician, who understood and agreed with the intervention.

PHYSICAL CRISES AND PSYCHOTHERAPY

Physical crises naturally take precedence over a psychotherapy session. This fact is frustrating for both the client and the therapist. The client who is not frustrated may be using excuses of physical problems as resistance, which can be explored. The therapist's frustration provides some taste of the feelings experienced by the client, who lives always with the possibility of a crisis and separation.

But we know that crises will occur. How can anticipation solve problems these crises present to the psychotherapy? The therapist may want to consider these options:

• Hospital visits, if only as a visitor to provide continuity and support.
• Home visits.
• Telephone support during hospitalization.
• Use of this time to provide consultation and support to family members and other caregivers.

The physical crisis is always a time for the client's reconsideration of vulnerabilities and strengths. Many return to therapy with new insights and new concerns. All are reminded of mortality. If opportunities for insight and change have been squandered, this is often recognized and new effort is put into the psychotherapeutic process. In some cases, of course, it will be up to the therapist to ask why the client has not introduced the topic of the new crisis, and to query about what emotions might underly this omission. In either case, the physical crisis provides new incentive and new material for the psychotherapeutic process.

For the psychotherapist, too, a client's physical crisis may raise feelings about one's efficacy and the role played in the client's life. Issues of vulnerability and mortality may be raised during these crises, and clinicians should use these situations to investigate their own fears and concerns.

CHRONIC SYMPTOMS AND PSYCHOTHERAPY

PWAs normally go through cycles of feelings of well-being contrasted with periods of fatigue and other chronic symptoms. But physical ailments, other than crises, are not barriers from psychotherapy, no more than they are for cancer patients and other physically disabled persons.

Sometimes a client, regardless of the difficulty of the disability, will make heroic efforts to come to the weekly session. One client, a former dancer who mourned the continual deterioration of his legs, would walk very slowly, with a cane, some five blocks for each therapy session. Others in similar situations often seek transportation from friends, from public systems, or ambulette services.

But in anticipation of these circumstances, the psychotherapist must know what means he or she is willing to use to spend time with the disabled client. Home visits or telephone sessions should be considered. Also to be considered are issues such as the practitioner's willingness to spend time with the client as he or she becomes more demented. If the client has personality changes or memory loss, will the practitioner still consider the psychotherapeutic relationship important? For many who believe therapy is a thinking process that involves working toward insight and behavior change, the work with a demented client may be frustrating, in that change or insight may not occur. It may then distill to a relationship of support and caring, without the "action" of goal-oriented psychotherapy. Can the practitioner continue this relationship of support, without frustration, impatience, or a belief that the client no longer requires "psychotherapy?"

Clearly, in the subspecialty of HIV-related psychotherapy, the clinician must conceptualize his or her role as being much broader than in other psychotherapies. Monitoring for physical and psychiatric disorders, as well as for other dangers such as suicide, cannot be neglected in the psychotherapeutic contract with an HIV-positive person. The therapist's willingness to act as an effective monitor is not only indicative of one's commitment, but also may have a significant effect on the client's well-being.

7
Neuropsychological/ Neurological Issues

It is inevitable that most, if not all, neurologists, psychiatrists, and psychologists will need to become involved in managing HIV-1 infected persons (World Health Organization, 1988, p. 24).

Alonzo lay in his bed all weekend, haranguing the nurses and complaining of rectal pain due to hemorrhoids. He did not want medicine forced upon him. When nurses insisted he swallow the pills while they watched, he refused his medications. He wanted to see his wife, but when she visited he was angry and hostile, driving her away. He would refuse to leave his bed. The hospital staff had made up its collective mind: Alonzo was a difficult patient, who received only necessary care and nothing extra.

When a psychologist first visited him, Alonzo would not put down his *El Diario.* Asked a question, Alonzo would pretend not to listen or understand. "Que?" he'd shout, time and time again. The next visit was with a translator, and Alonzo brightened and expressed himself in his native Spanish.

He explained that he was married three years ago, and had worked 11 years as a bus driver for a tour group. More recently, he began doing decorative ironwork, for which he seemed to have a knack. He would look at some decorative work and duplicate it well. Smiling, he recalled his talents and his financial independence. He added that he had been a professional entertainer many years ago in his native land, and that he had written music. He had a tape recorder by his bedside to play that music.

But there seemed to be little else he could recall. The year? He was several years off. And he was not interested in telling the month or day of the week either. He was in too much emotional pain, he explained. Too depressed, too tired, and what was the point of making an effort if the disease were to kill him soon anyway?

The diagnosis? Has Alonzo always been a difficult person, now exacerbated by organicity? Does Alonzo have a major depression, one that could be alleviated by tricyclics or by Prozac (fluoxetine)? Is dextroamphetamine (Ritalin) indicated? Does he have an agitated delirium or dementia, which may require Thorazine (chlorpromazine)?

And what is the prognosis? Can Alonzo regain his independence? Will he work again? Can he go home and be independent or will he require home care due to this condition?

Alonzo's case illustrates the extremely complex diagnostic and treatment issues raised by the neuropsychological aspects of HIV infection. He was found to have AIDS dementia complex. His memory loss was most notable. But he was also confused, apathetic, withdrawn, and regressed. Also, when he was most difficult, he likely was delirious and required medical treatment for that condition. He was no saint; a domineering person at home, he had alienated his now-adult children, and the behavior in the hospital was extreme. But he was no "scumball" either.

AIDS-RELATED DEMENTIA: PUBLIC CONCERNS

Much attention has been given to the complication of HIV now called AIDS dementia. With increasing research, the issue of AIDS dementia should become clearer. But whatever scientific evidence is available has not calmed the public's fears. The public is still concerned that men and women responsible for public safety—bus drivers like Alonzo, for example, airplane pilots, and police officers—may be driven mad by the AIDS virus and suddenly act irresponsibly.

The World Health Organization (1988) responded to those fears in a 1988 report: "There is no evidence that asymptomatic HIV-1 infected individuals pose special problems in safety related occupations" (p. 16). That statement is supported by much recent evidence, including a report by Selnes et al. (1990) who found no decline in neuropsychological test performance among 238 HIV-positive asymptomatic persons in the early stages of infection, compared to HIV-negative control subjects. Miller et al. (1990), in a study of 727 asymptomatic HIV-positive men and 84 symptomatic men, compared to 769 controls, also found no differences in functioning between asymptomatic subjects and HIV-negative subjects.

Clients too are concerned about AIDS dementia. Some say they will commit suicide if they believe they are losing their mental faculties and physical capabilities.

Statistics indicate that perhaps 40% of individuals with AIDS will show central nervous system (CNS) involvement (Price et al., 1988). In the Miller et al. (1990) study, while asymptomatic individuals had no neuropsychological differences compared to seronegative controls, symptomatic individuals as a group showed significant differences in performance on measures of short-term memory and of motor and psychomotor timed components compared to groups of asymptomatic and control subjects.

In about 10% of HIV-infected individuals, neurological signs are the first symptoms of AIDS (Levy, Bredesen, & Rosenblum, 1988). About 7.5% of AIDS patients reported to the CDC have reliably diagnosed neurological illness at time of diagnosis (Levy & Bredesen, 1988). Autopsy studies have found abnormalities in the brains of up to 65% of patients (Navia, Jordan, & Price, 1986).

Although neurological abnormalities are found in autopsy studies, it is unclear whether they evidenced themselves behaviorally. We do not know if every brain abnormality has a behavioral counterpart. Or, perhaps the patients died before AIDS dementia was demonstrated. The advent of new drugs, promising longer lives, raises an important question: Will increased longevity mean more PWAs will live long enough to have symptoms of dementia? Hopes are now invested in such drugs as zidovudine and other antiviral drugs that may attack the virus, possibly also diminishing AIDS dementia.

AIDS DEMENTIA DIAGNOSTIC SIGNS

Even before AIDS, organicity involving the central nervous system was understood as, basically, a five-fold syndrome which included impaired orientation, memory, intellectual functioning, and judgment, along with liability and shallowness of affect.

In AIDS, symptoms have generally been described to include:

1. In the early stages:
   a. Forgetfulness.
   b. Difficulty concentrating.
   c. Confusion.
   d. Cognitive slowing.
   e. Balance problems.
   f. Leg weakness (peripheral neuropathy).
   g. Apathy.
   h. Withdrawal.
   i. Dysphoric mood.
   j. Behavioral changes.
2. Later stage symptoms include:

a. Global cognitive dysfunction (in severe cases).
b. Slowed verbal responses or mutism.
c. Psychomotor retardation.
d. Wide-eyed stare.
e. Quiet confusion.
f. Indifference to illness.
g. Organic psychosis.
h. Peripheral neuropathies.
i. Incontinence.
   (From Navia, Jordan, & Price, 1986; McArthur, 1987.)

A staging system for AIDS dementia, included in a *Neurology* editorial (Sidtis & Price, 1990), lists stages 0 (normal functioning), 0.5 (subclinical or minimal symptoms), and 1 (mild symptoms with unequivocal evidence of impairment) through 4 (end stage, in which the patient is nearly vegetative). For other detailed discussions of HIV-related organic disorders dementia, complex, consult Brew, Rosenblum, and Price (1988), Elder and Sever (1988), Levy and Bredesen (1988), Navia, Jordan, and Price (1986), Perry (1990), Price and Brew (1988), and Tross et al. (1988). For a review specific to neuropsychology see Kaemingk and Kaszniak (1989).

Central Nervous System Involvement

With AIDS patients, HIV-related dementia was originally referred to as subacute encephalopathy or subacute encephalitis and then was called "subcortical dementia" (Navia, Jordan, & Price, 1986). The latter terminology was used to link clinical manifestations to anatomy. It is believed that HIV-related changes occurred first in the lower regions of the brain, including the brain stem, basal ganglia (bundles of nerves in the forebrain concerned with motor control and emotional behavior), and then in the white matter, known as subcortical matter (Navia, Cho, Petito, & Price, 1986). For comparison, recall that Parkinsonian symptoms, also considered subcortical, occur due to a dopamine deficit that can be traced to the substantia nigra, which is functionally related to the basal ganglia. And, compare that information to the amnestic "cortical dementia" symptoms of Alzheimer's patients, whose memory loss is related to outer cortex, or grey matter, changes. Interestingly, CAT scans of AIDS patients also indicate some cortical shrinkage, but it is still unclear whether any AIDS dementia symptoms are caused by this.

Kaemingk and Kaszniak (1989) noted that the cortical/subcortical distinction is controversial. The subcortical hypothesis of HIV dementia has some support, they wrote, but still requires prospective evaluation. Nevertheless, consideration of HIV dementia as "subcortical" provides a useful way of integrating information about symptoms and pathology, "a theoretical basis for developing hypotheses about brain–behavior relationships, a guide for neuropsychological test selection, and possible directions for treatment" (Kaemingk & Kaszniak, 1989, p. 322).

Peripheral Nervous System Involvement

Also common are peripheral nervous system manifestations, generically called peripheral neuropathies. There are two types, sensory and motor.

Sensory neuropathy is experienced as burning in the feet, toes, and fingers, and as decreased sensitivity to touch. Gait may be disturbed because the patient may have poor sensory feedback. Termed distal symmetric peripheral neuropathy, it presents usually in persons with fullblown AIDS, is associated with dementia, and indicates a downward course.

In contrast, a motor neuropathy, called chronic inflammatory demyelinating polyradiculoneuropathy, manifests itself earlier in HIV illness, primarily HIV-positive or ARC patients. Motor weakness is prominent; no sensory problems are evident. The muscular problems include bladder and bowel problems. The cause is demyelination, apparently caused by macrophages attacking and stripping the fatty sheath off nerves, including all cranial nerves except I (olfactory) and II (optic).

Other similar conditions may present themselves, the most common of which is Herpes Zoster, which attacks individual peripheral nerves and is extremely painful; skin lesions do not always erupt, and it remits spontaneously.

ETIOLOGY

The cause or causes of AIDS dementia have not been determined beyond doubt. Early researchers indicated HIV crossed the blood/brain barrier to directly infect the brain (for example, Ho, Pomerantz, & Kaplan, 1987; Shaw et al., 1985). Knowledge that the brain has CD-4 receptors, which enable the virus to dock on those cells, and the positive effects of zidovudine on some cognitive functions tend to substantiate that belief.

However, some studies suggest other organisms may also be at work. An intriguing recent finding was that of a research group at the U.S. Armed Forces Institute of Pathology. The group has reported finding evidence of a "virus-like infectious agent (VLIA)" later referred to as *mycoplasma incognitus,* in various tissues including the brain, of persons with AIDS (Lo, Shih, Newton, et al., 1989; Lo, Shin, Yang, et al., 1989). The authors conclude that "VLIA is a previously unrecognized pathogenic mycoplasma . . . [that] infects many patients with AIDS, produces fatal systemic infection in experimental monkeys, and causes extensive infection in previously healthy non-AIDS patients with acute fatal disease" (Lo, Shih, Newton et al., 1989, p. 598).

OTHER NEUROLOGICAL
OPPORTUNISTIC INFECTIONS

Several other conditions neurologically affect the patient with symptoms related to the location of the lesion.

Cryptococcal meningitis (crypto), the most common CNS fungal infection in AIDS patients (Brew, Rosenblum, & Price, 1988), affects the meninges, the tough connective tissue that covers the nervous system. Patients may have headaches, nausea, confusion, lethargy, or mutism. Treatment was very taxing until the experimental use and, finally, approval of fluconazole, an antifungal medicine now replacing amphotericin B as the first line of treatment.

Toxoplasmosis (toxo), caused by a protozoa, can cause focal neurologic signs, fever, headache, clouding of consciousness, confusion, and seizures. It is diagnosed by a blood test for "toxo titers," a CAT scan done after injection of a contrast dye, and response to treatment. Neurologists will examine the x-ray for focal lesions, which are surrounded by an obvious ring. About 5% to 15% of PWAs may have this condition (Price & Brew, 1988). It is treated by pyrimethamine and sulfadiazine.

Progressive multifocal leukoencephalopathy, a condition caused by a human papova(virus), JC, is called "multifocal" because there is selective demyelination in many areas of the brain's white (leuko) matter. Focal signs are evident, depending on the locations of the lesions. No proven effective therapy is available.

CNS lymphoma, a neoplasm, when large enough or deep in the frontal regions, can cause frontal or global symptoms.

DIFFERENTIAL DIAGNOSES
FOR AIDS DEMENTIA

Unfortunately, too many persons use the term "dementia" to describe transient conditions that may have nothing to do with AIDS dementia complex. The neuropsychologist must be more precise, and consider all possible differential diagnoses for whatever raises suspicions of AIDS dementia. Factors that point to other diagnoses include:

- Rapid onset of memory loss, which suggests delirium caused by an acute disease process or direct effects of acute organicity.
- Lateralization of neurological symptoms, including lateralized neglect, which indicates a focal lesion.
- Symptoms of delirium, characterized by rapid onset of clouding of the sensorium with waxing and waning of mental status.
- Aphasia. Rare in demented patients, it more likely results from cryptococcal meningitis or conditions which result in focal CNS lesions. Only in severe

cases, which have deteriorated to global confusion, are there deficits in language and visual perception, localized in grey matter.

Depression

Depression alone does not account for profound deficits. If depression is to be explored as a differential diagnosis, the recommended protocol includes neuropsychological testing to establish the current level of functioning, followed by a regimen of antidepressant medications, if not otherwise medically contraindicated. After a reasonable time to allow the antidepressants to take effect, a second neuropsychological assessment should be conducted. If there is no improvement or a downward trend in scores is obvious, dementia is the likely cause.

As part of the assessment, the examiner should also determine whether the client is responsive to prompts, as one would in an attempt to differentiate dementia from depression-related pseudodementia. Depressed persons are believed to be more responsive to prompts. Likewise, it is suggested that the depressed HIV-positive patient may be more responsive to prompting.

NEUROPSYCHOLOGICAL TESTING

The issue of whether to conduct neuropsychological assessment of an HIV-positive individual is similar to whether HIV testing was useful when no early medical interventions were available. Rex Swanda, PhD, a neuropsychologist at New York University Medical Center-Bellevue Hospital, suggests that the neuropsychologist consider whether the assessment will, on balance, be useful to the client, especially given the lack of treatment for HIV dementia (personal communication, September 1989). Situations in which neuropsychological assessment may be indicated include:

1. Assessment to provide an AIDS diagnosis so the client can receive social services and entitlements. According to CDC criteria for AIDS diagnosis, AIDS-related dementia alone can justify such a diagnosis. In some states, such as New York, the AIDS diagnosis, confirmed by a professional assessment, affects social services and entitlements.
2. To answer rehabilitative, self-care, or placement questions, such as: Can the person thrive in an apartment by himself or herself? How much supervision will be necessary? Can the client remember medications, appointments? What strengths remain? What rehabilitative strategies will be useful?
3. If significant problems are occurring, and physicians cannot attribute them to opportunistic infections or metabolic or other organic factors. AIDS-related dementia is not always evident from CAT scans or MRIs. Baer (1989), for instance, reports 18 persons who were "clearly clinically de-

mented" but "results from corroborating laboratory and radiographic studies were variable. On CAT or MRI, 12 patients demonstrated abnormalities (atrophy and/or white matter lesions), four had normal results on these studies and two had no recent study. On lumbar puncture, five had a non-specific abnormality . . . three had normal findings and 10 had no recent study" (pp. 1286–1287).

Other Considerations

The AIDS-related neuropsychological inquiry should include the following considerations:

1. Emphasis on therapy.

The neuropsychological evaluation—including the feedback to the client and caregivers—should be done as therapeutically as possible, Swanda of NYU-Bellevue suggests. The feedback to the client may in fact skirt the issue of a dementia diagnosis and focus instead on strengths and rehabilitation strategies for weaknesses.

2. Clarification of the presenting question.

Rarely does a physician or social service counselor articulate exactly what is required. This occurs because psychologists have failed to educate others about what can be accomplished through assessment. A typical presenting order may be, "Do some psychological tests and tell us if he can live alone." This hardly begins to describe what information you may need to provide. You need to know where the person will live (in familiar quarters or a new residence), is a kitchen involved, are grocery stores and other facilities nearby, to name just a few details.

Competency questions are often raised. Typically asked is the too-broad question, "Is the patient competent?" Again, this fails to state adequately the question. Competency is recognized as a situation-specific matter (Groves & Vaccarino, 1987). In this case, is the real question, "Is the patient competent to refuse medication?" Or is it, "Can the person live at home without assistance?" Specificity is required.

3. Consideration of the patient's age, education, employment, culture, psychological, psychiatric, and medical histories and current conditions.

Sidtis and Price (1990) also cautioned about the confounds of testing conditions, experience of assessors, length and intensity of testing, as well as past and present neurologic diseases and medications.

Is English a second language? What cultural factors may be relevant? Is the person very dependent? Or very independent? Is there a history of alcohol or other substance abuse, or could the client have used controlled substances recently? One clinician requires a drug screen before neuropsychological assessment. Could a psychiatric disorder be present? Is there an academic history that may indicate a preexisting learning disability or deficit due to head injury?

What other medical problems exist that may complicate the assessment? HIV-positive status does not rule out or override retardation, neurosyphilis, Alzheimer's, or other conditions that may also interplay.

4. Realization that no single instrument can lead to a conclusive diagnosis.

A diagnostic conclusion is the result of an interweaving of data from several different instruments. Norms for any specific test may be "inaccurate" and require interpretation only in light of other findings (see, for example, Trahan, Patterson, Quintana, & Biron's [1987] critique of the finger tapping test). Psychologists spend long semesters attempting to learn individual instruments and then fine-tune them into psychological testing batteries that are valid; that is, they are proven to assess what is claimed.

5. Diagnosing dementia.

A diagnosis of dementia can be obtained only with longitudinal testing, to confirm stasis or cognitive deterioration over several months. Consider the factors that may contribute to decrement or improvement in performance over time, including change in medical condition, introduction of zidovudine or other medications, and alleviation of depression.

Because psychological and cognitive testing requires specialized expertise, these tests should be conducted only by those with graduate-level training and certification. Most publishers of assessment materials, in fact, will not sell them to those who cannot certify special expertise. Assessment by someone not competent is unprofessional.

Instruments Used in Research

Among the groups using psychological batteries for research purposes is the Multicenter AIDS Cohort Study Neurological Working Group, including representatives of departments and schools at Johns Hopkins, Northwestern, UCLA, and the University of Pittsburgh (Miller et al., 1990; Selnes et al., 1990).

This group uses the Digit Span from the Wechsler Adult Intelligence Scale—Revised (WAIS-R; Wechsler, 1981); the Symbol Digit Modalities Test (Smith, 1982); Rey Auditory Verbal Learning Test (Rey, 1964); the Controlled Oral Word Association Test (Benton, 1968); the Grooved Pegboard (Klove, 1963) and the Brief Symptom Inventory (Derogatis & Melisaratos, 1983) and, in Los Angeles only, the Trail Making Test, Parts A and B (Reitan, 1979).

Clinical Batteries

More clinically oriented is Swanda's battery, which is intended to assess as many different areas of functioning as possible (personal communication, September, 1989). His battery can include:

- The WAIS-R (Wechsler, 1981). If a person is unable to respond to those tasks and the floor effect of the instrument may affect the result, Swanda will use the Peabody Picture Vocabulary Test (Dunn & Dunn, 1981) or, if necessary, Raven Progressive Matrices (Raven, 1960; see Lezak, 1983, pp. 502–505).
- Shipley Institute of Living Scale (Pollack, 1942), sold by Western Psychological Services. It is a 10-minute paper-and-pencil test that produces a "conceptual quotient" and an estimated "intellectual quotient."
- Rey Auditory Verbal Learning Test (Rey, 1964), which includes several learning trials of new words, providing the examiner with the subject's learning curve.
- Digit Span from the WAIS-R (Wechsler, 1981), both forward and backward.
- A cancellation test, in which the subject is asked to scan rows of numbers and indicate repeated numbers in each line.
- Finger-tapping, from the Halstead–Reitan Neurological Battery (Halstead, 1947).
- Grooved Pegboard (Trites, 1977).
- Trailmaking A and B. A perceptual set and speed test which resembles "connect the dot" tasks. Part A requires subjects to connect numbered circles and Part B requires a shift from numbered to lettered circles (Reitan, 1979). Reitan provides "cut-off times" that separate normal persons from those with organic problems. Miller et al. (1990) noted that Part B of the test "discriminated AIDS patients from controls in most studies of HIV-related encephalopathy" (p. 198). Persons with AIDS dementia not only exceed the cutoff times by large margins, but also may get "lost": They tend to forget the task, take indirect paths between circles, repeat themselves and make other strikeovers, fail to make easy shifts from one set to another, perseverate and otherwise indicate confusion.
- (Rey's) Complex Figure Test, which measures immediate and delayed recognition (see Lezak, 1983, p. 395–402).
- Benton Visual Retention Test (Benton, 1974). A 10-card series with three administration options (see Lezak, 1983, pp. 447–451).
- Word Fluency, in which the subject names animals and marketplace items. Norms are in Lezak (1983). Twelve items is the cutoff, with average production about 16 items. When writing down the subject's responses, Swanda groups the words by 15 second intervals, to determine if slowing occurs.

Another instrument, a well-normed cognitive battery, has been used with other neuropsychological tests at the Spellman Center for HIV-Related Disease, New York. The instrument is the Woodcock–Johnson Psycho-Educational Battery—Revised, Tests of Cognitive Ability (Woodcock & Johnson, 1989). Based on the Horn–Cattell theory of intellectual processing, it measures several AIDS-pertinent intellectual abilities, including shortterm memory and longterm retrieval, processing speed, and decision-making speed. Age norms are provided and subjects' achievement can be compared to these norms. The subtest tasks may be somewhat daunting for the moderately- to severely-impaired client. Calculation of scores is time consuming and requires assessor's attention to detail.

NEUROPSYCHOLOGICAL FINDINGS

Interpretation of neuropsychological findings should include comparing current to premorbid functioning, observing behavior during test taking, and relating the findings to the presenting problem. These are discussed below.

Comparison to Premorbid Functioning

Assessment requires accurate comparison of current functioning to premorbid functioning. The neuropsychologist should attempt to obtain high school transcripts with standardized test scores. If baseline information is unavailable, the neuropsychologist may wish to use the information provided by Matarazzo and Herman (1984) for estimation of premorbid WAIS-R intelligence quotients based on number of years of schooling. Using data from the WAIS-R standardization sample of 1,880 persons, the authors noted that the "relationship between years of education completed and measured intelligence is a stable one" (p. 632). Based on that, Matarazzo and Herman's (1984) data, reprinted in Table 7.1, allows a crude estimate of an adult's premorbid WAIS-R IQ. To arrive at the estimate, clinicians can use the mean years of education completed and their corresponding IQ values, or the correlations of coefficient. These inferences, the authors warned, "should be made sparingly and, then, only cautiously" (p. 634). If these tables are to be used, the clinician must also inquire about the qualitative nature of the client's education: whether the subject attended regular or special classes, number of years repeated and whether administrative promotions occurred, and reasons for dropping out, if that occurred.

Subjects with a history of intravenous drug use are difficult to assess for dementia because they may have had low premorbid functioning, learning disorders, or cognitive deficits that result from drug abuse and drug-related organicity. While it may be impossible to untangle the causes of very low

Table 7.1. Mean Verbal, Performance, and Full Scale IQs, by Age Group, with Means, Standard Deviations, and Correlation Coefficients in WAIS-R Standardization Sample (Matarazzo & Herman, 1984).

	AGE GROUP								
	16–24 (N=600)			25–44 (N=550)			45–74 (N=730)		
YEARS OF EDUCATION COMPLETED	VIQ	PIQ	FSIQ	VIQ	PIQ	FSIQ	VIQ	PIQ	FSIQ
0–8	82.9	86.1	83.0	77.3	82.5	78.4	88.8	91.0	89.0
9–11	97.8	98.7	98.0	88.4	91.5	88.8	96.8	99.5	97.6
12	99.0	98.5	98.8	97.4	98.6	97.6	103.6	103.0	103.5
13–15	108.8	106.5	108.6	105.2	105.4	105.6	109.5	105.2	108.2
16+	112.0	111.4	113.6	114.0	110.7	113.8	119.2	111.9	117.8
Correlation coefficient*	.39	.28	.38	.67	.50	.63	.66	.47	.62
Mean	99.4	99.5	99.4	99.5	100.2	99.7	100.3	100.0	100.2
Standard deviation	14.6	15.1	14.9	15.3	15.6	15.7	14.9	14.9	15.0
Means years education for age group:	11.4			12.7			10.8		
Standard deviation:	1.9			3.0			3.3		

*Years of education with VIQs, PIQs and FSIQs on the WAIS-R, by age group, for the standardization sample.
Copyright © 1984 by the American Psychological Association. Adapted by permission.

assessment scores from an IVDU, the scores can nevertheless be used to describe current functioning.

One instrument useful to describe current functioning is the Vineland Adaptive Behavior Scales (Sparrow, Balla, & Cicchetti, 1985), which assesses a person's communication, daily living, and motor skills. This instrument provides age equivalencies as well as percentile scores and helps to describe current levels of functioning. The Vineland has the advantage of task-oriented questions which can help the psychologist qualitatively describe functioning.

This assessment device suggests that a clinician also use inquiries regarding concrete living tasks. For example, a task for ages 13 to 15 on the Vineland is, "Use a pay telephone." The assessment subject can be asked to demonstrate use of a pay telephone, including choice of proper coin. Further, for our purposes, the subject can be asked what or who to dial in case of emergency (911, in many communities), and what to say to concretely describe the emergency, such as "someone lying unconscious on the floor." Other face-valid questions can be asked, depending on the presenting problem: how to cook a meal, how to shop, how to take medication and when, etc.

Behavioral Observations

Skillful behavioral observations of test-taking activity can be extremely useful. Difficulties with Trailmaking as well as with other pencil-and-paper tests help describe the client's functioning. Descriptions of pauses, memory lapses, tip-of-the-tongue phenomenon, and efforts to perform concrete tasks will contribute to a useful report. Also important are the client's reactions to successes and failures. Is the client indifferent or does he or she become increasingly distraught? Were certain tasks terminated prematurely? Why? What is the client's frustration threshold?

Interpretation Related to Presenting Problem

A conclusion specifically related to the presenting problem is essential, and is sometimes inadvertently overlooked. The referring sources' concerns and questions should be reviewed and responded to in the report's conclusion. Additionally, recommendations should be made for rehabilitation and adjustment to the current situation, both for the client and for caregivers.

COPING STRATEGIES
FOR DEMENTING CLIENTS

Clients who have a degree of dementia or are becoming blind due to CMV retinitis can benefit from training in coping strategies, as can their caregivers. Dementia, as noted, presents in many ways. While no special rehabilitative-type science has been developed for **AIDS** dementia, an extensive rehabilitation and care literature exists for other physical conditions, including Alzheimer's or elderly dementia.

Suggestions for helping a demented person include:

1. Maintain consistency of environment, including how family and friends regard the client, as well as the client's living situation.

This is not the time for changes in the patient's "system." If Aunt Rose invites the client for lunch monthly, this should continue. The patient's living quarters should remain stable, with foods kept in their usual positions in cabinets and refrigerator. (A chart of those positions can be posted, if necessary.) If the client keeps an orderly closet and dresser, that order should be maintained.

2. Creation and active administration of a "care team," which will help the loved one cope.

Team projects may include scheduled visitations, or assignments for regular telephone checks. The primary care giver could organize friends to call the patient, just to check and to provide reminders (frequency of calls is a judgment of family and the consultant). A fail-safe system should include the possibility of access to the living quarters if the **PWA** does not answer an expected phone call.

3. Reminder system.

Some clinics and doctors write appointments on business cards, but these too often are lost. Clients are encouraged to carry calendars and to note all appointments, or ask physicians' assistants and others to write the appointments into the calendar. Unfortunately appointments are missed because clients fail to consult their calendars. One useful tool is the oversized calendar, posted in the bedroom. The client is urged to transfer appointments from the calendar book to the oversized calendar, and to consult it daily or more often. Friends are asked to remind the client whether he or she consulted the calendar.

4. Adaptation of computer technology and easily available gadgets.

More technology is becoming available to remind people of appointments, and medications. One useful gadget is the pill box which can be set to beep at medication time. Other applications clients find helpful are subscriptions to a telephone service that will make reminder calls. Many well-known mail order catalogs advertise goods that, with some creativity, can be used by a neurologically impaired **AIDS** patient. A recent Hammacher Schlemmer catalog included an alarm clock with a three-inch diameter alarm shut off button, which can be used by those with motor neuropathies. The catalog also has a clock that projects the time in 3-inch high numbers on the ceiling, for those with movement or eyesight problems, and a talking pocket watch, made by Seiko, which has a synthesized voice to announce the time. Also, several companies and other groups provide information on disabled persons' use of computers (see Appendix).

5. Reality orientation.

Some who have serious dementia may remain socially appropriate but are not oriented to place, time, or circumstance. One hospital patient, awaiting placement in a skilled nursing facility, greeted his visitor by saying he couldn't stay for long, because he had to be at work in 10 minutes. As with the elderly, it is suggested that friends and visitors continue to orient the patient to time, place, and circumstance.

6. A safe environment.

This includes monitoring of the person's condition and a willingness to call the physician if any changes occur. This also includes surveying the person's living quarters and removing or locking up any dangerous substances.

7. A realistic outlook on support.

Family members and other caregivers must be realistic, both to themselves and to their loved one, regarding what they can provide. Too often, a caregiver will castigate himself or herself for becoming fatigued, irritable, for wanting a respite, for fantasizing escape or, even, the patient's death. These are natural feelings that accompany caring for a chronically ill and debilitated person. These feelings are exacerbated when a caregiver, for whatever reason, fails to seek respite or otherwise take necessary time off.

Caregivers must realistically assess what they can provide, relative to the type of services the PWA requires. Little is accomplished and all suffer if the impossible is attempted. Consultation with the patient's physician, social worker or case manager may introduce options, such as longterm care, which may be perceived as abdication but which, in the long run, may benefit all.

8

Consultation/
Case Management Model

As AIDS is redefined as a chronic condition, the focus of attention broadens "from medical status alone to functional ability, since functional level is the key to understanding the consequences of chronic illness and to defining the need for services" (Benjamin, 1989, p. 146). The objective of keeping someone at the highest level of functioning "can be achieved to the extent that a comprehensive, *coordinated* [italics added] continuum of services is available," Benjamin noted (p. 147).

A consultation/case management model is suggested as that coordinating mechanism. This model has two overlapping components: The first is consultation, which is primarily provision of specialized information and psychoeducational services to clients, caregivers, health care providers, and others in the community. The relationship is short-term; no long-term psychotherapeutic relationship is contracted for. The second is case management, which entails interdisciplinary linkage and coordination of services.

Both the means and the end of this model is *integration*. In the provision of consultation and case management services, one integrates HIV expertise with other specific psychosocial and community knowledge and provides a creative and useful amalgam. In case management especially, one strives to integrate many different systems: family, neighborhood, the larger community, health care, and other service providers.

Use of this model extends the range of the psychotherapist's services, making for more effective utilization of one's body of knowledge. The model enables mental health practitioners to utilize on behalf of their clients that which they have a wealth of: Access to community resources and information, intra- and extracommunity contacts, insight into the interplay among systems and the savvy to use these for the client's benefit. Social workers, specially trained in case management, traditionally have made the most advantageous use of this information on their clients' behalf. Those in other professions have sometimes squandered their knowledge and other resources by shying from consultant/case management approaches.

Of course, case management may trouble some traditionally trained persons concerned with boundary issues within the context of psychotherapy. Yet, several different applications of the model are possible: within a flexible conceptualization of the psychotherapeutic relationship, based on one's training, the therapeutic contract, and the client's needs; or in nonpsychotherapy arrangements in which the clinician provides what are clearly short-term consultative and case management services.

Use of this model has great potential benefits to the client, caregivers, and society. The practitioner using this model addresses concrete HIV-related issues both for clients comfortable in a psychotherapeutic relationship as well as those either not interested in or not likely to benefit from traditional psychotherapeutic modalities. Families and friends who care for an HIV-positive person are often in great need of consultation services, which can range from simple education, such as infection control, to highly technical, such as neuropsychologically based rehabilitative-type advice. Moreover, consultation services can be provided to other professionals, such as internists and general medical practitioners who may be familiar with medical aspects of the illness, but not with some of the psychosocial aspects; attorneys; substance abuse program staff; and other mental health practitioners.

While only empirical studies can determine the actual benefits and cost savings of consultation/case management models, HIV-related applications may promote earlier and better use of prevention information and services, including those involving substance abuse; increased compliance with medical regimens; reductions in service duplication (such as that produced by patients' undetected "hospital hopping"); decreased inappropriate use of medical services, such as emergency rooms; better "fit" between needs and services, and decreased or more appropriate use of entitlements due to higher functioning. Some foundations and government agencies are already testing different case management models.

This chapter will briefly review the consultation and case management roles, and then address more specifically the functions, goals, and other concerns the practitioner must consider.

CONSULTANT ROLE

The specific aspects of the consultant's role are limited only by one's ability to make creative applications of knowledge, and the willingness of the community to take advantage of specialized information. By knowledge is meant not only HIV-related knowledge; in fact, various aspects are fairly widely known, at least in professional circles. What sets the individual practitioner apart is his or her ability to mix HIV knowledge with other specific psychosocial information. For example: Many clinicians may understand, in generalities, substance abuse issues, especially as they regard HIV. But a psychologist or clinical social worker who has experience with a community's adolescents may be able to recommend substance abuse and HIV prevention strategies that speak to the specific needs of those teens.

The consultant's role, then, is to take specific information in several realms—HIV, psychosocial functioning, community mores, among the many possibilities—and offer useful and sensible advice, interpretations, and applications.

To individual clients, the private practitioner and institutional staff member alike may provide information about community medical and social service systems; systems coordination; and HIV infection, including transmission, prevention, and ethical issues. Many clients do not know enough to ask the proper questions; the consultant empowers clients to ask those questions, and to obtain improved services. The consultant may also help the client deal with such difficult issues as: "I am going on a job interview. Should I tell them I have AIDS?" Or, "I told my dentist I was HIV-positive and he told me he wouldn't see me anymore. What can I do?" Under these circumstances the consultant may choose to articulate certain principles ("Would you tell a potential employer that you have diabetes, or a seizure disorder?") or make referrals to legal service agencies or other appropriate professionals. As the clinician gains expertise and contacts, these other professionals become more accessible and this accessibility is lent to your clients.

In such institutions as hospitals and community mental health agencies, the mental health practitioner can also have an important consultant's role regarding HIV. Psychiatrists have a medically related consultation–liaison function within hospitals. The psychosocial, nonmedical consultation–liaison role can easily be filled by psychologists, especially those cognitively behaviorally trained, social workers, and others. As nonmedical personnel prove their clinical and economic benefit, institutions will more quickly realize that the medical model cannot solve nonmedical issues such as the sociopolitical, psychosocial, and spiritual aspects of a patient's life.

Conceptualizations of clients' issues in biopsychosocial, rather than strictly medical, models are already being used in progressive hospital settings. Montefiore Medical Center's family practice residency program employs social workers and psychologists not only to train the residents in behavioral medicine, substance abuse, family systems, and AIDS, but also to provide consultative services in community clinics. Also at Montefiore, Peter A. Selwyn, M.D., a family physician, has received federal funds for his efforts to integrate primary care and substance abuse treatment, with emphases on HIV and family.

For the psychologist who serves as psychosocial coordinator of that integrative project, an illustrative consultation is that provided the wife of a man on methadone. She considered methadone a drug that should be avoided, and wanted to know more about methadone detoxification and AIDS prevention. The consultant requested that she return with her husband so they could discuss the situation and the roles of methadone maintenance, including AIDS prevention. While that practitioner was to provide neither case management nor traditional psychotherapy, his consultation was to help alleviate misconceptions and reduce family stress.

Finally, clinicians sometimes overlook the opportunity to interpret and explain the needs of their clientele to the political, legal, health delivery and other systems in the community. Consultation is not only for the individual and caregiver. So the community can better understand and serve HIV-positive persons, clinicians must also consult to city councils, community boards, boards of education, courts and other legal agencies, and community groups.

CASE MANAGEMENT ROLE

Another clinical role is that of case management, important in both the private practice and institutional settings. A private practice client who has minimal or inadequate social support or is becoming debilitated may require case management services to improve quality of life. In the institution, a case management system may wisely utilize mental health professionals to coordinate services.

What does case management encompass? Again, the field is limited only by one's creativity, sense of service and ethics, and one's professional comfort with providing these services. A psychiatric nurse may provide counseling, liaison with a mental health agency as well as a primary care provider, and may also help coordinate home care and entitlements. A psychologist may assess the resources—cognitive, financial, social—of a client and then coordinate a program of care with caregivers and other agencies. A case manager may want to telephone clients to remind them of appointments; empower them to be more forceful with health care providers; discuss prenatal care with a pregnant client and her partner; help the person comply with drugfree programs. The essence, of course, is integration across disciplines and improved care.

Why a psychotherapist? It may be that the psychotherapist has the longest and deepest relationship with the client and, in the absence of an active family member or other caregiver, best knows the client's needs and desires, as well as what the institution or community can provide. The psychotherapist may be the best person to integrate an individual's needs with the realities of community resources. Should it always be the psychotherapist? No. The psychotherapist may not desire that role or, if a client's service problems are primarily medical, others in the institutional or community systems may be more appropriate case managers.

GOALS

When taking a consultation/case management stance, the following goals should be considered:

- Client safety.

All advice, information sharing, communication between systems, is dedicated to the client's well-being.

- Consideration of what the client desires.

The client is, after all, the employer. The client may not easily or readily articulate desires; but it is the clinician's task to learn them.

Two aspects are involved: The first is consideration of the premorbid personality and its effect on current goals. If the patient has shown no interest in risk-taking before becoming ill, it is unlikely this should be a case management goal. The second aspect is the determination whether client desires are realistic. Both caregivers and clients may over- or underreach. The consultant should be able to provide both an assessment and well-considered information to enable setting and attainment of realistic goals.

- Empowerment of the client.

Especially in the consultant mode, the goal is to provide the client with power and autonomy. The clinician's task is not to harbor a regressed patient in a sick person's role, either by inappropriate overinvolvement or by supporting another caregiver's overinvolvement. A long-range view of the consultation/case management model should always include empowerment as a goal through such means as education, political involvement, and legal recourse.

- Empowerment of natural caregivers.

As the situation requires more case management, there may be a tendency to consolidate power and remove it from other caregivers, if only to expedite matters. As with the client, one goal is to empower caregivers, so they can better utilize resources. The task is coordination and management, not autocratic rule.

- Improvement of quality of life.

This is the optimal goal.

- Maintenance of stability.

Stability is crucial for everyone, but particularly so for a person whose chronic illness makes him or her feel out of control. The practitioner's task may be to ensure the stability of the client's situation, either directly by case management or indirectly by consultation to caregivers. Stability provides a message that events are in control.

- Discerning and providing structure.

Is there structure, a "holding environment," that ensures the client's safety? Determine who cares for the client, who makes decisions (and if these are different persons, the reason), and who is responsible in a crisis. Besides family, naturally occurring structures include day treatment programs, hospital-based care programs, and methadone clinic programs that provide counseling. If no secure structure exists, the professional's role may be to seek a structure in a community agency or hospital, or to provide some temporary structure.

- Use of the least restrictive environment.

Among professionals' responsibilities are difficult judgments about clients' living conditions. Concern regarding the least restrictive environment often arises with clients experiencing cognitive difficulties. A more restrictive environment may make the task easier for caregivers, but the primary responsibility is to the client. The consultant/case manager may help caregivers to understand the tasks of helping a demented PWA (see Chapter 7) or may suggest care by a home health care agency instead of institutionalization. Alternatively, the consultant may help the caregivers deal with guilt feelings if institutionalization is the least restrictive environment.

- Monitoring overmedicalization.

As noted, persons with HIV infection inevitably are drawn into a medical subculture. The medical model, however, cannot successfully address all HIV-related problems, which include family systems and emotional, spiritual, and other nonmedical aspects. The consultant may serve to remind parties that holistic care, which includes medical approaches but not to the exclusion of other concerns, may better serve the HIV-positive person.

- Shoring up the situation, especially in a crisis.

If the practitioner has adequately discerned the situation, no crisis will be unmanageable. However, if a crisis does occur, or if someone enters therapy in crisis, the first goal is to shore up the situation.

- Anticipatory management of changing needs.

This again recapitulates a theme of this volume—that the practitioner must be sufficiently competent and AIDS-aware, both generally and in particular to the client in order that few surprises will occur. Needs will change, which is not necessarily problematic. However, these changes should be anticipated.

• Assistance with bureaucracies.

Depending on the community, bureaucracies can be relatively benign or an unimaginable quagmire. Unfortunately most learn about bureaucracies after hard knocks and mistakes. Organizations that may be involved with HIV-positive clients include those that govern Social Security and disability (including private coverage) and other entitlement payments, housing services, medical services, and medical insurance carriers.

• Services for caregivers.

Caregivers are often ignored as attention is focused on the medically ill person. Often caregivers unrealistically assess the limits of their energy, and focus on caring for the HIV-positive person to their own detriment. Professional service providers may also ignore those caregivers. The consultant may want to refer caregivers to support groups, refer them to their own psychotherapists (to avoid conflicts of interest), or include them in a family therapy with the HIV-positive client, with the goal of improving their situation. In some cases, family members may realize the limits of their endurance and want to change the caregiving structure; for instance, parents may want a debilitated son institutionalized. To assuage their guilt and validate their needs, they may seek a consultant's "permission" for the alternative plan.

• Consideration of and referrals for legal documents, including wills and powers of attorney.

Legal issues vary from state to state regarding form, format, witnessing, enforceability, and other legal aspects. A power of attorney may be characterized as "durable" or "medical" and is used especially when the client wants someone other than the "next of kin" to make decisions. By signing a medical power of attorney, the client allows the person designated to make medical decisions, if the client cannot make them. In states without laws requiring doctors or hospitals to respect these, generally the wishes of the patient are nevertheless acknowledged. A consultant should stress the importance of obtaining legal advice regarding these documents *before* they are needed. Some AIDS-related community groups provide workshops and inexpensive legal assistance in writing wills and powers of attorney.

• Clarification of issues regarding "do-not-resuscitate orders" and living wills.

These are documents in which the client states what type of medical interventions he or she would prefer. The legal weight of Living Wills is different from state to state. DNRs, signed in the hospital, generally have great weight. These documents have temporal considerations: A young person may want all efforts at resuscitation if there is the possibility of a long life. A mortally ill PWA may choose to sign a DNR order declining resuscitation attempts.

PERSONS INVOLVED

If we conceptualize the HIV-positive person's situation as medical, psychological, social, familial, political, and so on, then the hierarchy of the medical model is inadequate to the task of either empowering the client or ensuring the client's holistic welfare.

The case management model provides a different view of the client's many systems. In this, the systems are interactive: The transportation system is necessary if the client is to be treated by the medical system; the social service system must be reckoned with if benefits are to be received. No system is paramount and none stands alone without the aid of the others. This reframing is necessary if we are to treat all aspects of the client.

The case manager's role, too, must be reframed as one that empowers the client, and derives its power from the client. The case manager must take a cue from the model: The systems are equal, and the players are collegial. That, of course, is an ideal, and one often encounters turf and status issues among practitioners. With skillful practice, case management may supersede these barriers so clients may be better served by all the systems.

With AIDS-related work, case management takes on added complexities. Many more systems and many more persons may be involved in a PWA's care than, say, that of a cancer patient. If one did not know better, it would be easy, for instance, to overlook an ophthalmologist or, perhaps, a nutritionist.

The following professionals should, typically, be involved in the care of an HIV-positive person:

- Physician, either in private or hospital-based practice.
- Neurologist, when nervous system disorders are manifested.
- Ophthalmologist.

CMV infects the retina causing loss of eyesight, but experts believe the damage can be halted. An HIV-positive person should have regular ophthalmologic checkups, preferably every 6 months, according to Steven Teich, MD, a New York retinal specialist (personal communication, November, 1989).

- Pulmonologist, when respiratory disorders, such as PCP or TB, occur.
- Infectious disease specialist.
- Hospital system personnel.

If the client has been hospitalized, a hospital social worker or other professional may be providing postdischarge planning or case management. If none is provided, a social worker nevertheless may have been responsible for obtaining services during hospitalization.

- Nonhospital social service agencies.

These may include AIDS-dedicated community groups, disability- and welfare-dispensing agencies, city or state agencies, depending on the locality. In New York City, a client may be enrolled at the hospital's social service department, an AIDS-related organization such as Gay Men's Health Crisis, a city agency that provides a caseworker, and Social Security offices.

- Pharmacist.

Because the pharmacology for an AIDS patient is so complex (and expensive), contact with a knowledgeable pharmacist is indispensable. Medications, including zidovudine, can be quite costly. Some pharmacies provide discounts to PWAs.

- Dentist.

Some dentists shun HIV-positive persons, yet sometimes the first manifestations of HIV-infection are in the mouth. Some communities have specialized dental clinics for HIV-positive persons. A network of private practitioners willing to work with HIV-positive persons is generally known by AIDS-related community groups.

- Spiritual adviser or clergyperson.

The spiritual aspects of the client's life may become more important or receive greater consideration now.

- Occupational therapist (OT).

Early in the epidemic, a PWA was left without additional services such as OT. Now, a dedicated OT can help prepare the client for chronic illness.

- Physical therapist.

A competent physical therapist can aid physical fitness and ambulation, especially important due to neuromuscular complications and the inactivity during hospitalizations.

- Nutritionist.

Diet is often considered crucial to HIV-positive persons. However, many have come up with radical ideas regarding diet. A certified professional nutritionist or dietician can contribute to the client's general well-being.

- Home care agency.

If home care is being provided or anticipated, the client may have a nurse or other professional managing the case through the agency. Home care may include visits or shifts by professionals ranging from attendants to specially trained registered nurses. Services range from basic help with bathing through "high tech" nursing that includes intravenous infusion of medication, such as Ganciclovir (DHPG), or perhaps nutritional supplements. Home care for PWAs is part of the next decade's medical care picture because of its low cost compared to that of hospitalization.

- Psychologist.

Trained in assessment, behavioral medicine, and neuropsychological assessment, a psychologist may be used to help with neurologic dysfunctioning, rehabilitation strategies, and health-oriented psychotherapy.

- Family.

Even though family members may be nonsupportive or distant, they need to be included in the case management picture. Some, relying on the legal aspects of familial ties, appear at crucial moments and severely question or attempt to take over management of their relative's care. To overlook them early in the illness is to do an inadequate job of managing the client's resources.

- Primary caregivers.

Generally it is useful to think of one family member or caregiver as primary, and enlist that person in the client's welfare. Many PWAs, especially gay men, are likely to have a primary caregiver other than a blood relative. If a primary caregiver is other than a family member, it is important to have clear whether this person is legally empowered—through a power of attorney or other legal instruments—to make decisions on behalf of the client.

Do not be left with the impression that a competent consultant/case manager can integrate all aspects of an HIV-positive person's care into a smoothly running system. Many stumbling blocks exist—including personalities, familial dysfunctions, turf rivalries, and poorly functioning social service systems. The goal, however, is not perfection. It is improvement in the client's care. Consultation and case management models have great potential in providing cost-effective, improved client care.

PART 3
THE THERAPIST'S FEELINGS

9
What the Therapist Brings to the Session

Billy was the one client the therapist could not touch. A man with severe erythemous dermatitis, his face looked as if he had walked wet through a sandstorm. It was not sand covering his face but flaking skin. His eyes were deep blue, and when he began to cry during the therapy session it appeared as if an oasis pond suddenly overflowed, with a rivulet coursing across a parched desert floor.

Severely swollen, Billy's arms looked like pink sausages in transparent casings that couldn't hold the contents and were cracking. He could hardly move his fingers. When the crying began, the therapist reached for a tissue and handed it to the patient, but Billy's fingers could not grasp it. The therapist awkwardly tucked the tissue between two fingers and sat down again. He said goodbye before leaving, but did not shake hands, did not touch the patient on the arm. This was someone he referred to another counselor.

Among the ways that HIV-related psychotherapy is different from other psychotherapies is the extent and depth of the feelings that surround and are evoked by HIV. Many flee from any aspect of HIV or AIDS, many react angrily, many blame the victims. While these persons may have the luxury to flee or to rail against groups and individuals, the psychotherapist who is asked to enter into a relationship with an HIV-infected person must be more reflective. Those professionals who can admit homophobia, anger with drug users, or irrational fear of AIDS, and who reject supervision or information that may change their feelings, may decline to work with HIV-positive persons; we should acknowledge their honesty and encourage additional insight. Of more concern are the clinicians who may have unexplored covert and subtle feelings that can color the therapeutic relationship, damage the client, or be a source of self-recrimination for the clinician.

Apart from anger and prejudices, all persons have unexamined areas dealing with death, abandonment, and existential fears. The psychotherapist who experienced abandonment, who may be HIV-positive, or who has other unexplored anxieties brings these, too, to the relationship.

These unexplored areas are of great importance because, no matter what the type of therapy, the clinician hears and otherwise experiences the client through his or her own feelings. Moreover, the client experiences what is truly the psychotherapist, no matter how we pretend otherwise. Silences reveal as much as words. The shifting in the chair or the quick blink of the eye is meaningful to the client and is carefully watched. So, if psychotherapy rests on the therapist's ability to care genuinely for the client, then the therapist's ability to care genuinely for the HIV-positive client rests on the ability to acknowledge, confront, and understand fears, angers, and prejudices. No shame should attend to having these feelings; the shame is in conducting psychotherapy without self-examination.

If the frontier of psychotherapeutic work is the practitioner's attention to his or her own feelings, then HIV-related psychotherapy may be the most difficult of frontiers. This chapter will first discuss the ubiquity of prejudice, and will then focus on concepts of countertransference, and subtle and unsubtle preconceptions brought to sessions with HIV-positive clients. An exercise, using a list of inquiries regarding HIV-related psychotherapy, concludes the chapter. The following chapter, 10, discusses how the client and the situation may provoke feelings. The final chapter in this section, 11, discusses self-care for psychotherapists who work with HIV-positive persons.

IRRATIONAL FEARS, COVERT PREJUDICES

> I've had people say to me, "Thank God for AIDS. It takes care of the blacks, the Puerto Ricans, and the homosexuals." I can deal with the people who say that because their prejudice is overt. It's the subtle prejudices that are hard to deal with, and I think each of us needs to look at the prejudices in ourselves when caring for persons with AIDS. ("When caring," 1987, p. 1)

Caregivers, including therapists, are representative of society and in no way immune from the irrational beliefs and prejudices relating to HIV that are so much a part of our communities. These fears regarding both those at risk for AIDS and the virus itself are well documented.

A survey (Douglas, Kalman, & Kalman, 1985) of 37 medical house officers and 91 registered nurses, using a homophobia measure, found a mean score at the low end of the homophobic range. About 10% of respondents agreed that gays who contract AIDS are "getting what they deserve" (p. 1310).

Twelve of 37 physicians (32%) and 27 of 91 nurses (30%) agreed that respondents "feel more negatively about homosexuality since the emergence of the AIDS crisis." Feelings regarding HIV-positive drug users often are expressed in such phrases as "Why bother?" (Batki, Sorensen, Faltz, & Madover, 1988).

Exploring irrational fears of AIDS, Wormser and Joline (1989) asked medical professionals who had just heard a lecture "that clearly emphasized the routes of HIV transmission" (p. 181) whether they would eat cookies prepared by a person with ARC. Overall, 32 of 45 respondents (73%) said they would not. In a group given a scenario in which a leukemia patient offered the cookies, 20 of 43 (49%) said they would not eat the cookies.

FEELINGS AS "COUNTERTRANSFERENCE"

That the psychotherapist has feelings regarding the client is beyond argument. To label those feelings "countertransference" is to enter into an area that even the psychoanalytic community continues to debate. However, it may be useful to conceptualize feelings regarding clients in two categories, as Muskin the psychiatrist and analyst, suggests (personal communication, July, 1989).

He notes that psychodynamic psychotherapists recognize two types of countertransference, generally: The first can be characterized as "broad spectrum" reaction to a client. It includes irritation, titillation, anger, feeling manipulated, feeling opposed, or feeling easily acquiesced to. These are immediate indicators of how the client deals with the environment, and are necessary and useful parts of the therapy. Using the feelings evoked by the client, the therapist can recognize how the client is regarded by others, and how he or she regards those in his or her world. One way to conceptualize these is as "what the client brings to—or injects into—the therapy."

The second countertransference is "narrow spectrum," which involves the therapist's feelings that are idiosyncratic perceptions of the client, distortions based on the therapist's psychodynamic history. An obvious example is the therapist's reaction to a client who reminds her of her Uncle Ned, who was coarse and crude. The client may be coarse and crude, but may be many other things which are obscured by this narrow spectrum countertransference. Another example of this type of countertransference is a reflexive response—such as hostility—to certain types of clients. For example, while some therapists are reflexively hostile or uncomfortable with psychopathic personalities, others find them appealing. These narrow spectrum feelings, products of the therapist's emotional make-up, are counterproductive in psychotherapy because they introduce extraneous matter into the relationship.

When applied to HIV-related work, therapist's feelings may include romanticizing, at one extreme, or disparaging of HIV-positive clients, at the other extreme. Positive feelings may result in an increased desire to be helpful, or too much involvement without allowing the client to be responsible and autonomous. Conversely, negative feelings may result in a stance that holds the client to inappropriate—or, perhaps, unrealistic—standards of responsibility and is, paradoxically, denigrating and demoralizing. Subtle negative feelings, as well as positive feelings, may also make us overly responsible for and overinvolved with HIV-positive clients.

These feelings cannot be avoided. Rather, acknowledge that HIV-related therapeutic work can be both more emotionally volatile and more emotionally subtle, and take steps to become aware of emotional responses. When one feels a need to be tougher, with the client or oneself, one must be aware enough to ask why. When the practitioner feels angry and hostile, he or she should ask why.

This self-scrutiny should not involve judgments about one's own and colleagues' predispositions and reactions, any more than one should judge clients. It is curious that although psychotherapists encourage others' self-scrutiny, they are sometimes very reluctant to explore themselves. Many are reluctant to seek out supervision or peer discussions because they fear others will judge them; their reluctance, too, often stems from self-judgment. Should the therapist who could not touch the client be judged and found wanting? Or should he or she be comforted and the pain, awakened by the client's plight, understood? Perhaps clinicians should first acknowledge that they bring to HIV-related psychotherapy a terrible judgment of themselves, as well as expectations, fantasies, and fears of incompetence.

EXPECTATIONS

Therapists always have expectations for their own performance, and for that of the client.

Weisman (1981), writing about cancer caregivers, observed that caregivers in sustained relationships provide the promise of "safe conduct," which may include information, choices, availability and a pledge that the caretaker can be counted on. But, Weisman also noted that the caregiver expects something from the client in exchange: gratitude, cooperation, remuneration, recovery, and other responses that depend on the idiosyncratic needs of the caregiver. Feelings for the client may depend on how readily the client fulfills the expectations created for him or her.

A therapist's feelings also may depend on how he or she construes the meaning of "safe conduct." If it is understood as rescue including, subtly, rescue from chronic illness and death, the therapist may become depressed, demoralized, and angry as the efforts seem to fail.

The complexities of HIV-related psychotherapy make the possibility of these types of disappointments almost certain for the unaware psychotherapist.

For Ourselves

A clinician's failure to live up to his or her own performance expectations, many of which are very subtle, can quickly demoralize someone working with HIV-positive clients. Among these expectations are those regarding the emotional requirements to do this work, rescue fantasies, and the efficacy of concrete plans,

Tough Enough?

One common belief regarding the emotional prerequisites for working with HIV-positive persons is that one has to be "tough enough" to deal with those who have chronic illness and who will, in the final stages, die. This misconception is built on the belief that one handles difficult issues (living, dying, and death) by building a suit of armor and hiding within.

To believe that one must be tough enough is perhaps the first and most deadly of misconceptions, one founded in defensive emotional responses to issues of living and dying. In fact, if one is "tough enough" then one cannot conduct psychotherapy with anyone, let alone with this special group. To be tough means the practitioner is also inaccessible—unable to experience another's feelings because of a decision not to experience one's own.

The subtlety of this issue is indicated by the very clever reasons given for not being emotional with, or for, clients. One therapist told his supervisor that a client nearly brought him to tears, which he fought back so that he could be strong for the client. The supervisor suggested that perhaps the client did not need a show of strength that would indicate that the client was "weak" in comparison. Rather, perhaps the client needed empathy and the connection of shared tears, which was the therapist's genuine, but stifled, response.

Another caregiver's subtle denial of emotional response was expressed this way: "I told him that his sister had died last night of AIDS. He cried, but I didn't. I think the sister is in a better place, she's not suffering anymore." That stance, that the deceased is at peace, does comfort. But perhaps it also denies the clinician's feelings of loss. Another, possibly more accurate, statement is that one felt a mixture of sadness from the loss, as well as comfort with the knowledge that the deceased is suffering no more. One can cry and feel relieved for the person who died, both without embarrassment.

Does anyone really want a therapist who cannot empathize and respond genuinely, who cannot show fear or sorrow, sadness or joy? Clients choose humans for therapists, rather than computers, to be with, to feel resonation, to feel understood.

Rescue Fantasies

Rescue fantasies, which can be very subtle, are the surest route to a sense of impotence and burnout (see Chapter 11). Two rescue fantasies are common in this psychotherapy: The first regards the physical, that somehow one can contribute to a cure. While everyone hopes that a cure will be forthcoming, and some believe that elements of psychotherapy (such as stress reduction) may lead to greater longevity, a psychotherapist would not tell a client that the therapeutic relationship will contribute to physical cure. And, it is doubtful that any practitioner would admit to believing that the relationship is physically curative. Yet, at some subtle level, there are practitioners who may have the fantasy that they can contribute to physical healing. In the face of physical decline, the fantasy is disproved, and they feel impotent and powerless.

Another rescue fantasy is the belief that the therapeutic relationship may create significant lasting personality changes that will contribute to an emotionally healthier dying. The best example is the hope that a person with a narcissistic or psychopathic personality disorder will, through psychotherapy, not die as he or she lived, but move beyond the psychopathology to a "healthier" death. Several situations militate against this: First, it is unlikely that persons with personality disorders will enter AIDS-related psychotherapy with goals of personality change. That may be the therapist's goal, born in rescue fantasies. More likely, the client's goals will be more situation-specific. One HIV-positive male with a borderline personality disorder entered psychotherapy only after his arrest, and his goal was to have the therapist intervene with the criminal justice system. Less-disordered clients may have goals that have nothing to do with long established problems, but enter because they are suffering acute stress from the HIV condition; they may terminate when the stress is relieved. For some, a tranquilizer is as good as a relationship.

The predictable response to unfulfilled rescue fantasies is a sense of helplessness and impotence, blamed on the therapist's inabilities, rather than on impossible expectations. With feelings of helplessness and impotence, the clinician targets himself or herself as, at best, having failed this client or, at worst, being generally incompetent. The result may be that the therapist feels dispirited and demoralized but is unable, without self-awareness, to attribute this to a desire to be powerful in the face of AIDS.

Belief in the Efficacy of Concrete Plans

Many therapists attempt to help the client produce some concrete proposal for action, a "homework" to be begun or accomplished before the next session or within a reasonable time. Success, then, is measured by behavior and noncompliance is "failure." These concrete plans may indeed help a client to deal with problems, produce a product from the session, and may break inertia and give some impetus. This type of therapy is often indicated and its appropriate use is to be applauded. A danger lies in a practitioner's subtle belief that therapeutic efficacy is gauged by the amount of concrete response. If response is not forthcoming, grave disappointment in one's ability to produce behavior change may occur.

One other consideration regarding concrete planning is suggested by Tunnell (1987), who argued that psychotherapists who pursue active problem solving may be attempting to avoid their own feelings of helplessness and anger.

> As long as the *patient* has a plan to avoid the adversity and negativity of life, he won't have to deal with feeling helpless. As long as the *therapist* has a plan to avoid dealing with the patient's adverse situation and negative feelings, he or she won't have to deal with feeling helpless in the therapy hour. (p. 4)

The therapist should be cognizant of why problem solving is being attempted, and explore whether the attempt serves to reduce therapist anxiety.

Therapist's Life Situations

The therapist also brings elements of his or her own life into the therapeutic relationship. These may include:

• The therapist's own HIV status.

McKusick (1988) noted a case in which the therapist is HIV-positive, and described the concerns regarding disclosing the seropositivity to the client. These situations are always highly idiosyncratic, and no general guidelines can be provided other than that the client's needs are paramount. Supervision is clearly indicated.

• Therapist's experience of loss and abandonment.

This may affect the bond with the client, especially at times of physical crisis.

• Feelings regarding own's own sexuality, including homosexuality.
• Feelings regarding sexuality and vulnerability of relatives, including one's children.

McKusick (1988) describes a therapist's protectiveness regarding a dating-age daughter as a countertransferential issue.

Expectations for the Client

The bottom line is, many practitioners subtly expect clients to behave as the practitioners do. When clients do not, clinicians are sometimes surprised and often angry. The clinician may then recover and attempt to explain the discrepancy, but always in terms that, although polite, make it clear that the client has failed to live up to "standards." Of course, there *are* reasons: Psychopathology makes a person act "badly," or the client is influenced by a subculture or is a "victim" of some sort. Nevertheless, the client is usually judged relative to a baseline of mainstream good health and sense. If the client is offensive, different in some way that intrudes on a practitioner's beliefs, then that therapist may become angry.

An example of caregiver anger occurs in urban emergency rooms that treat intravenous drug users. Staff there may become angry with patients who are treated, released, and then return because they fail to comply with medical instructions. These patients are perceived as deliberately defiant and irresponsible. With caregivers' (unrealistic) expectations affronted, the staff become angry.

Therapists too become angry when clients do not fulfill expectations. More self-aware or guarded, therapists may use words other than "angry:" surprised, saddened, confused, to name several. But each is in reaction to behavior that is unexpected. If we expected it, we would not be angry, surprised, saddened, or confused.

We bring several other expectations of clients, including the following categories.

Expectation of Noncompliance

The therapist, especially one who works with HIV-positive clients out of a sense of social duty, is likely to regard them with a great deal of compassion. However, accompanying compassion and sympathy may be the subtle belief that the HIV-positive person is a martyr, and that such a status exempts the client from conformity with accepted standards of behavior, either inside or outside the therapy room, or from efforts to reach therapeutic goals. Some clients, especially those with an exaggerated sense of entitlement, may contribute to this perception.

The danger in romanticizing the client as a victim is that this obscures a clear view of whatever reasons prevent the person from formulating and working toward psychotherapy goals. Reasons that inhibit success may be rational and valid, but they require a nonbiased assessment.

The issue of goals and behavior was prominent with Sandy, a former teacher who engaged in weekend drinking binges. His physician made it clear that the drinking binges had to stop because they jeopardized him in many ways—physically, emotionally (they exacerbated a depression), and financially. Sandy was defiant: The binges were his only pleasure, and he would not stop. How was his psychotherapist to respond? Does the therapist confront the client regarding the self-destructive behavior?

One may argue that Sandy's life is short, and he should be able to enjoy a few pleasures. Another argument is that a confrontation will make Sandy wary about the psychotherapy, and it is better to have him appear weekly, despite his binges, than never. Another view is that the binges are entrenched behavior and efforts to end them will end in defeat. Should we impose expectations on this tragic man?

The issue of how to confront Sandy is a matter of personal style and training. But the question that pertains to the therapist's feelings regarding a PWA is this: Would these arguments be used to avoid confrontation with a nonHIV client? Why would an HIV-positive client be treated differently? If Sandy were a woman, or a pregnant woman, how would she be treated?

A therapist should understand why he or she would choose to give an HIV-positive client a less energetic or less confrontational psychotherapy. Making a victim out of the client may be one reason. Another reason for a therapist's reluctance to confront self-destructive behavior may be symptomatic of subtle devaluation of the client, or a signal of the therapist's despair, which may reflect the client's hopelessness.

Attractive Clients

Not dissimilar is the special treatment—in the straight and gay worlds alike—often accorded the physically attractive client. The positive feelings and expectations they invoke may obscure a clear view of their circumstances. They may also make a therapist reluctant to press and confront, as one would other clients.

A sad situation unique to these clients may occur with their physical decline. If the therapist's attachment to the client is at least partly due to physical attraction, what will be his or her reaction to the end stages of HIV illness? The therapist must be very conscious of the bases of positive feelings, and not abandon this client when the attraction diminishes, either out of disappointment or despair.

Overidentification

One does not have to be gay or a drug user to identify with the client. Identification can be positive: It provides empathy, and conveys warmth to the client. The alternative—failure to identify—indicated by empathic failures or an inability to provide a warm and caring environment is at best off-putting, and at worse rejecting. Overidentification is more subtle and yet more obvious. The therapist who overidentifies not only observes and empathizes with the client, but is unable to separate himself or herself from the client. The therapist becomes ineffective because he or she can no longer observe objectively. The therapist is not able to distinguish himself or herself from the client, and can no longer exercise the judgment of a distinguished observer.

Whether gay men are the better psychotherapists for gay men is a related issue. The answer is, "It depends." As with any therapy, the efficacy of the client–therapist match depends on personal needs and characteristics. Some gay men find more comfort and empathy in psychotherapists with the same sexual orientation. Further, these psychotherapists may be able to act as role models in a way that a heterosexual person cannot. If a client can benefit from a role model, then a match of sexual preferences may be useful. However, other gay clients may benefit from a heterosexual therapist. A male therapist's sexuality is often raised by the gay male client who is struggling with his relationships with the straight world, and particularly his father whom he may have experienced as rejecting. If the therapist suggests immediately the possibility of discomfort with a straight therapist, the client is allowed to enter an area of concern that may be central to his relations with the straight world. John, a 30-year-old gay male, immediately responded to this inquiry by talking about his relationship with his father, and the father's perceived inability to empathize with his gay son.

12-QUESTION EXERCISE

Prominent among the deep and extensive feelings that are aroused by HIV issues are those concerning death, pain, abandonment, God, family, and other matters of great importance. Although persons of sensitivity and insight may acknowledge that these issues are crucial, they seldom consider them until confronted. Others, anticipating these issues, fear they will freeze and not be able to respond appropriately. In psychotherapy with HIV-positive persons, we are likely to be confronted with these issues.

In seminars, I ask participants to examine their feelings regarding these issues by responding to several very difficult but common questions voiced by HIV-positive clients. At first, I conceptualized this as a psychotherapy exercise to help therapists anticipate and prepare their psychotherapeutic responses. But the exercise seems more useful as a way to examine psychotherapists' feelings.

In this exercise, I ask that you take each question and first respond as you would if it were asked by a client in a session. Perhaps you could get a colleague, supervisor, or friend to read them to you, and respond, even if only by jotting down a note. Then, go through the questions a second time and respond honestly, as you really feel. Then note the disparities between the two responses.

This exercise is useful in several ways: It helps the therapist to hear what response would be given initially to the client, and to understand what feelings provoked the response. This response, including the spoken or unspoken emotional response, is likely to reveal our fears, hopes, leanings, and other personal issues that could interfere with an authentic relationship. For instance, did the therapist resort to technique because of anxiety? Second, an examination of the differences, if any, between the immediate response and the more honest response bear examination. Our more thoughtful response may tell us how we really regard these issues. Third, the honest response and the differences can be grist for one's own psychotherapy, analysis, or supervision. Finally, the exercise does allow one to anticipate and plan for these questions in sessions.

It is better to have examined oneself through the exercises and, if necessary, decide not to conduct therapy with HIV-positive persons, than to enter into an inauthentic relationship, that is easily betrayed.

1. Why me?

What is your gut response? Is it, "Because you went out and shot up drugs"? Or "Because you were promiscuous and had anal intercourse." These are variations of "Because you did not follow the rules." The converse is, "Those who followed the rules did not become infected." All these statements carry a value judgment that is likely to affect the therapy.

Few practitioners said to the victims of Toxic Shock Syndrome, "It was because you used a tampon." This question, for the therapist, raises the issues of blame. Are Toxic Shock Syndrome and AIDS similar? What responsibility does one have for contracting an illness? And, to extend it, what responsibility does one have for one's having practiced unsafe sex, especially before there was knowledge of risk factors? And what are your attitudes regarding drug use? Is drug use a symptom of a personality disorder, and is a person responsible for his or her personality disorder? Are environmental factors to blame?

One consideration here is the therapist's concern with rules and social norms. Is the therapist a rule-follower, and uncomfortable with those who are not? Is the therapist angry with those who flout convention?

2. Will I die in pain?

This may raise anxiety because you do not know the answer, and are unfamiliar with medical responses to pain. Some persons, most noticeably intravenous drug users, report low thresholds of pain. Yet, these are the persons physicians seem less likely to treat for pain, because they fear being manipulated by patients who want to obtain drugs. What are your attitudes regarding pain control, generally, and pain control for persons who have abused drugs? Are you the kind of person who will not take a Tylenol, and hold others in contempt for "overmedicating?" You know persons have different experiences of pain, but are you open to that realization with the person in front of you? Are you willing to learn about pain control, generally, or whether AIDS patients actually die in pain?

This is the first of several questions that concern fears of dying. Have you thought of what you fear in dying?

3. Will I die alone?
4. Will you stay with me until the end?

Question 3 is a subtle form of question 4 and, in its subtlety, the request to the therapist may be lost. When asked in the form of Question 4, a direct plea is voiced. At one level, it may be asking, "Will you abandon me as others have, or as I fear others will?" At another, it may be inquiring, "Will you be by my bedside, and see me through this journey?" Practical and emotional issues interplay in your response to this question. Practically, your response could be dictated by the terms of the therapeutic contract, which was based on your careful assessment following the guidelines of Chapter 4. Also, practically speaking, your hospital visits to a client who may be deteriorating will be dictated by your schedule. If your August vacation were planned, would you change it if your client were dying? The emotional issues are very subtle and in many shades of grey, and these deserve careful analysis. Yes, your schedule is busy, but couldn't you get to the hospital? If so, what stopped you? What fears of loss and impotence may be at the bottom of your inability to "stay with me until the end?" These questions ask how close you can be to your client, and how much loss you can tolerate. If you find it hard to tolerate loss, do you disparage yourself and, possibly, the client? Will you allow yourself to explore this issue?

On the other hand, however, is the "caretaker" in you being manipulated? What is behind your eagerness to stand by and hold the client's hand? This eagerness should be examined, because it may indicate a grandiosity or rescue fantasy that can debilitate the therapist. Consider the possibility that your overinvolvement is in reaction to negative feelings. What might these be? Would your answer be different depending on the client's sex or risk factor?

Is it the function of the therapist to be at the bedside?

5. Can you stand to look at me?

Honestly, can you stand to look at the client? To touch him or her? Many become marked with Kaposi's Sarcoma (KS) lesions. KS also may cause severe swelling in some patients. Arms may be as big as logs, faces may swell and eyes close up. How necessary is it for you to have a client who appears attractive or normal? Is there a fear of disfigurement, or beliefs that scars run deep? What emotions are felt when you close your eyes and imagine being with someone disfigured?

6. Wouldn't you kill yourself if you were me?

This is one of the most difficult questions, and one of the most provocative. You should be clear regarding your response before you start therapy with HIV-positive clients.

The question touches on your beliefs in quality and quantity of life, and your despair and optimism. Some, such as the Hemlock Society, argue eloquently for the individual's right to commit "rational" suicide. Others will say that no suicidal ideation is rational, that it reflects a severe psychiatric disturbance, no matter how thoughtful the client appears. Which do you believe?

Would you be willing to collude in an AIDS patient's suicide, if you are certain you will not suffer professional repercussion? Or, are you convinced you would intervene to prevent a suicide, under any circumstances?

If you are convinced you would intervene to block a suicide, do you provide an informative statement at the beginning of therapy, to wit, "And if you should ever be perceived as in danger, I would have to act to ensure your safety." Or do you believe such a statement could bring the reply, "Sure, I'll talk to you about all aspects of my life, except for my consideration of suicide." Do you want to cut off the possibility of that discussion?

Further, while we may have some religious or ethical considerations regarding suicide, we may be confused about whether to apply these in therapy. One therapist, working with a Catholic patient considering suicide, may attempt to dissuade him or her by raising the issue of mortal sin. Another practitioner may feel more comfortable steering clear of religious issues.

And, to get back to the question, would you kill yourself in this situation? Do you reveal that to the client?

7. As I can't be cured, wouldn't it be better to give up?

Do you believe a person's life, even a dysfunctional person's life—a paralyzed person's life, or a murderer's life, for example—requires as costly and complete medical attention as your life? Is each life equal to the next? Or, is there a subtle ledger sheet that ranks different persons differently? If you believe in rational suicide, would you fail to intervene with a passive suicide which may involve noncompliance with medical regimens, signing out of a hospital against medical advice, or refusing to seek emergency treatment? Failure to intervene may involve not asking certain difficult questions because you would rather not hear the answers. Failing to ask or otherwise act is rooted in your feelings regarding this issue.

8. Is there a God?
9. Why would God put me through this?

In therapist and client alike, the asking and responding to this question raises profound questions of life's meaning and possibilities of connections with larger realities. This is the same question that arises during any tragedy. In the face of tragedy, can we believe in a benevolent deity? What role does the concept of God have in our lives? Is he or she a rescuer, or a fellow sufferer whose divine presence gives us courage? If God is a rescuer and we are not rescued, are we undeserving?

Responses to the client will be obviously influenced by the therapist's beliefs, the perception of the client's beliefs, and by community standards. If you believe in a punishing or vengeful deity, it is well to examine how this affects your feelings about the HIV-positive client. For a discussion of spiritual issues, see Chapter 16.

10. Am I forgiven?

Forgiven for what? And who is it that eventually forgives? Are you in a position to offer forgiveness—legitimately, as a clergy person, or illegitimately, as a mother or father figure? In yourself, do you bear hard feelings against the client or the person who infected the client? Does the client appear to be reacting to these feelings? Do you need to be forgiven for some of your feelings regarding the client?

11. What will happen to my family?

This question can raise feelings of punitiveness in the therapist, due to a sense that the client may be responsible for his or her own plight and, especially, the plight of family members, including children. Therapists who have lost parents or friends due to perceived "carelessness" may have difficulty empathizing with a person who has been careless about his or her health and therefore has "caused" others' suffering.

12. Why should I tell anyone?

Therapists should have their stance on this issue thought out. Does one believe, universally, that no secrets should be kept? Or can there be exceptions? Why should someone tell a family member who has always been rejecting? Is there a disparity between the therapist's goals for reunion and communication and the client's goals?

What is your reaction to the person who insists on maintaining the secret, although others may be injured? What of the man who continues to have unsafe sex or share needles, thus spreading HIV? What about the HIV-positive woman who chooses to bring the fetus to term, with the possibility that the child may be HIV-positive? And what is your stance on warning the partner?

These questions are not meant to provoke self-criticism or negative feelings. Rather, they should facilitate discussion and self-exploration and allow clinicians to anticipate and better respond to the client who raises these questions. Few persons have reason to consider these issues before being faced with them. Now, however, faced with these issues, we owe it to ourselves and the clients to consider carefully what we bring to psychotherapy sessions.

10
How Events Affect the Therapist

There is no reaction among patients that cannot also occur in caregivers (Weisman, 1981, p. 165).

I find myself become increasing anxious as my client, a dapper 50-year-old man who has traveled the world, continues to tell me that all is well, and he is without a care. I find myself shifting uncomfortably as he talks; the broader his smile becomes, the more unconvinced and uncomfortable I feel.

About 6 months earlier this man found himself in the hospital with salmonella sepsis, and now he had little memory of how he got there. As often occurs, he was reluctant to get help despite increasing fever and illness. A visiting friend found him dehydrated and delirious and called an ambulance. Three months after discharge, this client began therapy when a hospital social worker found he was inattentive to details concerning his illness and downright argumentative regarding his condition.

At the outset, he said he was not convinced about his HIV status, and requested another test. The second test, promptly provided, confirmed the first result. His doubt, after 3 weeks in an AIDS unit, was an early indication of his stance regarding his AIDS—one which was to become more rigid as he became more forgetful.

Early in his outpatient medical care, he was given zidovudine. But he argued that the medicine's purpose and regimen were never fully explained. Given a nebulizer for pentamadine, he later charged that no one taught him to use it. This scenario was oft-repeated: Each time medical staff were accused of having failed to address his problems, and he was angry. But each time they had, and the patient continued to swing between anger and blissful unconcern for his situation. I shifted uncomfortably in my seat with each statement of how splendid his situation was. I was experiencing his unexpressed anxiety.

Jonathan was another client whom I became very fond of during one year of work. In therapy he talked insightfully about his relationship with his father and his relationship with the church in which he had been raised. Although he had a relative in the ministry, Jonathan felt brave enough to picket a church he found unresponsive to his needs. In time, he became ill and was brought into the hospital with several opportunistic infections, including PCP and cryptococcal meningitis. Upon admission and for several days thereafter he had high fevers, could not speak, and had altered mental status. I watched him linger for several days and in desperation began combing through his medical chart. I believed, hoped, that something had been overlooked, that perhaps the weekend house physician had neglected an important test or failed to prescribe the right medication. I asked the head nurse to review the chart and offer a suggestion, which I could then take up with the physician and, if necessary, with hospital administrators.

Then suddenly, I drew back and saw myself for what I was being: a desperate family member watching a patient fail and feeling out of control. There had to be an answer that would allay my anxiety, and if only the answer could be found, then the situation would be remedied. I felt out of control, as do families in hospitals throughout the world. I searched for clues, for missed opportunities, for a second opinion. But no alternatives were available.

Each case illustrates feelings evoked in the psychotherapist by the events of HIV illness. This phenomenon seems linked to the emotional intensity of the experience of HIV-related illness, and facilitated by the caregiver's emotional links to the HIV-positive persons. Carolyn Moorhead, a registered nurse and analytic psychotherapist, in as-yet unpublished speeches, calls the phenomenon "parallel processing" when health care staff members' feelings mirror what the patient is experiencing (Moorhead, 1989). She finds this common with nurses, who spend the most time with the patients. No words are necessary in this subtle communication between patient and caregivers. Feelings are communicated by context, shared beliefs, nonverbal cues, all of which may evoke shared fears. One example, which is perhaps too simplistic, is that the staff's hopes soar when the patient's mood and outlook improves, and they become demoralized when a patient becomes depressed.

The psychotherapist, too, is affected by this mysterious process. As noted by Weisman (1981), who studied cancer patients and their caregivers, "There is no reaction among patients that cannot also occur in caregivers" (p. 5). The feelings of the HIV-positive client are often experienced by the therapist as his or her own. These include anger—at fate, medical caregivers, and others— and feelings of desperation, helplessness, fear, and despair.

I believe this phenomenon differs from Kernberg's (1984) conceptualization of projective identification. This occurs when a client unconsciously projects feelings such as hostility onto the therapist while trying to induce that reaction. The therapist unconsciously identifies with the projection, feeling hostile in response. The client then experiences the hostility being projected, fears the person under the influence of the projected impulse, and attempts to control the therapist now under the influence of this mechanism (see Kernberg, 1984, for a brief, understandable description). In the case of parallel processing, no projection occurs. Rather, the therapist resonates empathically with the client's plight.

This chapter will describe various manifestations of how the emotional experience of the HIV-positive person is evoked in the psychotherapist. The therapist's recognition of this phenomenon is important for several reasons: First, the recognition aids in understanding the client's emotional experiences (which perhaps cannot be expressed orally) under the stress of HIV. Second, the recognition helps the therapist to understand that these evoked feelings are normal during the psychotherapy and present opportunities to learn, rather than reasons to worry. Third, understanding of this evocative process will enable the clinician to better tolerate these negative feelings, heading off feelings of helplessness in the short run and burnout in the long run.

THE AIDS DREAM

Very often, the first startling emotional experience reported by a caregiver of someone who is HIV-positive is the AIDS dream. A remarkable occurrence, this is seemingly ubiquitous, reported by almost every caregiver intimately linked to a person with AIDS. Nurses and physicians new to a hospital AIDS unit or a psychotherapist with a new HIV-positive client report the dream within a matter of weeks. Typically, the dreams include being diagnosed as HIV-positive or with AIDS, or having a loved one, such as spouse or lover, similarly diagnosed. Reports of these dreams include feelings of dread, anxiety, panic, and other feelings sometimes too profound to be easily put into words. While terrifying, these dreams provide valuable empathic insights into the client's emotional state. They show us the terror and link the therapist's humanity to the client's. The dreams do not indicate unhealthy overinvolvement or evidence of the clinician's shaky emotional state and should not frighten one away from HIV-related psychotherapy. Rather, they invite us into its richness and mark a start of the process by which we confront our fears and grow, just as the client will.

OVERPOWERING NEGATIVE FEELINGS

The AIDS dream may leave us sleepless and disturbed, but we know it is ephemeral. However, in the reality of daylight, the client's negative feelings can overpower the therapist. This occurs especially when the client is in an unrecognized psychiatric crisis or when negative affect is extremely powerful.

One example was in the challenge of Kathy, who over several sessions intensified an attack on her therapist, saying he was useless to her, unable to help and uncaring. She had no previous psychiatric history, but was becoming so agitated that the therapist referred her to a psychiatrist, who initially prescribed an anxiolytic. A depression ensued, and Kathy was first put on Prozac, which was found to be too activating, and then nortriptyline. During the sessions of greatest intensity, the client's challenge to the therapist became more strident: You are no good; I do not know why I come to you. I am increasingly anxious (depressed) and you will not help me. At least the psychiatrist gave me medication, although that is not working either.

In the face of such a powerful expression of the client's feelings, the therapist began to lose confidence in his effectiveness. Could he *really* be useful to this client or was the relationship a fraud, he began to wonder. In the face of the emotional onslaught, the therapist begin to believe that the patient was correct, that he *was* ineffective. When the patient became more confrontative about the goal of the therapy sessions, the therapist, in his anxiety, found it difficult to express the goals and to articulate his role in attaining them. Bewildered, the therapist sought supervision and learned how he was overpowered by the client's negative feelings, which were about loss of hope and inability to focus on goals. The therapist, too, lost hope and sight of the goal, and this blocked him from saying, "No I cannot cure you, but I can help you to come to terms. That is why we're here."

Psychotherapists are not helpless in the face of AIDS. They can help the client live a better life, attain goals, come to terms, and confront dying and death. But often feelings of helplessness, spoken or not, are communicated in the psychotherapy session and evoked in the therapist, resulting in a therapist's loss of faith in himself or herself. The antidote is recognition that the loss of direction and faith is a product of the client's hopelessness, and redirection through supervision.

PRESS OF TIME AND THE FIVE STAGES

Another feeling the client may evoke in the therapist is frustration, which comes from a perception that despite the brevity of time and crush of therapeutic work to be done, the client is wasting time both inside and outside of the therapy room.

This sense of frustration may be worsened by some notions that the therapeutic agenda, perhaps the hidden agenda, should be to move the client through Kübler-Ross's (1969) five stages of terminal illness—denial, anger, bargaining, depression, and acceptance—as expeditiously as possible, and that failure to do so represents a therapy failure or, worse, a "bad death." The therapist then proceeds as if, "We need to reach anger by noon; acceptance by 9 P.M." When the patient seems unwilling to move through any therapist-dictated paces, the clinician who focuses on product rather than process may begin to doubt his or her efficacy or the client's capacity to attain (the therapist's) goals. Actually, it is rare that a person moves through all five stages, especially in the reported order (Schneidman, 1983). Some persons never reach acceptance; for others, what looks like denial may in fact be acceptance. The therapist should be aware that any striving toward programmatic goals may indicate the therapist's needs, rather than the client's. Frustration with the client may actually turn to anger which, if not recognized and understood, can jeopardize the therapy. The client is angry enough at fate; now the therapist is angry too, seemingly at the client.

Gerard, a man with KS, was entirely casual about psychotherapy throughout most of the final year of his life. Yes, he had the money for new shoes and shirts but no, he didn't have subway fare for his psychotherapy session. We're running out of time, we're running out of time, his therapist was feeling, as she saw Gerard falter. It was not until 3 weeks before his death that Gerard called the psychotherapist, and asked her to come by the hospital for a talk. The call was an indication that, to Gerard, the process of relationship, rather than the clinician's goals of product, was ultimately important.

Gerard and other clients who fail to hasten their steps in response to the call of mortality do not fail to act because they are ignorant of the facts, even when those facts are nakedly, and perhaps sadistically, spelled out by a frustrated and angry therapist. The client knows very well the facts of life; the press of time is even more real, frustrating, and enraging to the HIV-positive person. Gerard countered that frustration and anger with denial and avoidance but those emotions nevertheless "leaked" to the psychotherapist who became, likewise, frustrated and angry but who misattributed her emotional experience to the client's perceived recalcitrance. In fact, the therapist was experiencing parallel processing. Yet the misattributed feelings were so disconcerting that they temporarily blinded her to the client's obvious defenses and she failed, for a time, to make the necessary interpretation.

DEMENTIA AND PHYSICAL DETERIORATION

One disconcerting aspect of work with AIDS patients is the possibility of gradual physical deterioration, such as that caused by wasting, and cognitive deterioration. Those who are close to the PWA may see gradual changes in the person's appearance or cognitive acuity. A PWA may lose a large amount of weight over time, become weak and begin to look frail. At its worst, AIDS dementia can rob the client not only of memory but also of personality.

Many persons, friends, family, and psychotherapists may have strong feelings in reaction to the deterioration of the individual. These may include sadness, regret, anger, even aversion—any of which can lead to avoidance. Avoidance is the behavior that often signals underlying therapist distress. Any beginnings of avoidance should be flagged, the emotions that underlie it faced and understood, and the avoidance rectified, if possible.

With the therapist's sophistication, this avoidance can be cloaked in plausible reasons for reducing the number of therapy sessions or terminating the relationship: The client is too weak; or, the client's cognitive functioning is poor, making the PWA a poor candidate for psychotherapy. In the situation of an avoiding therapist, we have a parallel of the noncompliant client who misses sessions: The therapist will want the noncompliant client to explore reasons for avoiding therapy. The therapist who seeks to avoid the physically deteriorating client will also want to explore the emotional reasons for avoidance.

The exploration of the therapist's reaction to this phase of HIV-related illness may focus on fear: fear of the unknown, fear of what the deterioration represents, and fear of such deterioration in oneself. Discomposure in the face of cognitive deterioration may be especially understandable in those who have built lives and careers based on their intellectual capacities. These professionals may find themselves impatient with the cognitively distressed client, as they might be impatient with themselves under similar circumstances.

The exploration may also focus on one's own experiences with relatives, for instance, who have become physically ill or demented because of old age, Alzheimer's, or other debilitating condition. The avoidance that is aroused by physical and cognitive deterioration may also be a foreshadowing of the avoidance that comes with the client's dying.

AS DEATH NEARS

In psychotherapy we serve the living, but we cannot avoid the anxiety that attends to thoughts of death (Becker, 1973). While death is the ultimately predictable event, the moment of death is unpredictable during the course of AIDS. As death approaches, and perhaps withdraws again, therapists and all others in the client's family may feel more helpless.

It is during the last months of life that the client, and the therapist, may experience great difficulties maintaining the relationship. The client may be hospitalized and severely ill, perhaps not recognizing the therapist or not having the stamina for visitors. The therapist may experience anxieties that are new. This is a time for introspection and supervisory discussion, with a careful monitoring of reactions to the impending loss.

Client's Distancing

This man was skin and bone, walking with the help of a cane. He talked of increasingly ferocious battles with his roommate, physical deterioration that was very troubling, and how he was bothered by so many friends who would stop by his apartment—constantly it seemed—to check up on him. He wanted time alone, to clean his house, do his grooming. He'd rather not entertain others, he said. And he had a message for his therapist, too. These weekly psychotherapy sessions were also time-consuming intrusions into his life. He said he needed time to walk to the grocery store, to shop, and just to be with himself.

The therapist's first reaction was that grocery shopping surely cannot be as important as the weekly therapy hour. And how is it that he does not want friends to stop by anymore? Was it depression? No, he wasn't depressed. The clinician made tentative inquiries about distancing, and the client remained adamant that he just wanted time to do his chores, and to enjoy the doing. Ultimately the therapist chose to make no more queries or interpretations, and to accept the client's decision. He invited the client to call again in a few weeks, if he wanted to, for another appointment. Soon there was another hospitalization, for several HIV-related conditions.

In supervision, the therapist fretted that he had not been able to form the necessary bond that would have kept the client engaged in therapy. He said he felt inadequate. The supervisor suggested, however, that perhaps to this client the therapeutic relationship offered a sense of freedom: to leave, to return, to do the errands before death, unencumbered by appointments and the "musts" of a rigid frame. The therapist was not necessarily inadequate, but generous in his ability to open the relationship to the client's needs.

The client never returned home from that hospitalization, but he did call the therapist several times, and there were a few hospital visits. The therapist was able to communicate his regard for the client.

Sometimes, in the flickering moments, the therapist is not acknowledged. Perhaps the impending death is not acknowledged either or, secure in the therapeutic relationship, the client pursues a personal agenda. During a vacation, I was telephoned and told that one client, with whom I had a brief but fruitful relationship, was close to death. I travelled to the hospital to say goodbye, and found a man who looked far from death. He was chipper, smiling, sitting up in bed, and talkative. He said he had moments of confusion but was feeling better than he had in a long time. He seemed not to realize how close the doctor believed he was to death. After about five minutes, a nurse entered and announced another visitor outside. The client said he didn't want to miss that visitor, and waved me away, thanking me for stopping by. Thirty-six hours later he died.

As hard as it is to gauge when death will come, it is equally fruitless to gauge your worth to the client by the client's behavior in the dying moments. You have helped the person to the threshold. The client moves across it as his or her own abilities allow.

Therapist's Distancing

Seravalli (1988) wrote about the reaction of a physician to a dying patient. "With the worsening of my father's condition, the physician stopped being friendly and warm; his visits became rare and brief; his manner became quite detached, almost angry" (p. 1729). It is suggested that physicians may become angry because the patient's dying contradicts their healing skills. The therapist too may become upset and angry, for any number of reasons, and separate subtly from the patient.

Any subtle distancing from a very ill client should be explored in supervision or one's own therapy. Many plausible reasons and excuses may be offered: the press of schedule, the impossibility of geography, and the need to adhere to therapeutic frames, among them. But while some or all these may be involved, these reasons are often smokescreens for emotional issues. The therapist should explore existential issues. Some clinicians may acutely feel anxiety raised by issues of abandonment or death. Others may feel guilt, believing that they have not done enough, or powerlessness, believing erroneously that they can do nothing now.

Saying Goodbye

I have asked others, "How do you say goodbye?" When I leave the hospital on Friday, what do I say when I am not sure the patient will still be alive Monday? After many deaths in a hospital, and many suggestions by others, the situation still concerns me and still makes me feel anxious.

One mental health practitioner, who seemed to believe candor, however sadistic, is a higher value than gentleness, told a client, "I'm going on vacation and won't be back for two weeks. The doctors don't think you'll live until then, so I'm saying goodbye." This is not a recommended approach. Regard is not expressed by cold expressions of dubious "facts."

It seems now that a good farewell, when nothing is predictable, is a statement of regard in the present tense. For example: "It is always good to see you. It is good to talk with you and work with you. I learn a lot, sitting by your bed, and we share many emotions." The present tense expresses feelings of closeness, and does not end the relationship. Now, before departing, I sometimes use the message provided me by a loving client, who said, "I'll see you when I see you."

Afterward

The sad side of hospitals is how they respond with routine to death. Too often I arrive on Monday, to be told almost casually, "Mr. Jones, Mr. Smith, and Ms. Ruiz died over the weekend." For many health service providers, the three disappeared one weekend and are only briefly considered again. This happens again and again, to those in institutional settings. Rather than have people disappear in death, we need to stop, assess our anxiety and loss, and be with these individuals again. Seravalli (1988) suggests

> What a help it might be if physicians were to spend a few minutes in the room where a death has just occurred trying to find a place for it in their personal

and professional lives. Perhaps if we opened ourselves to what can be understood of the particular world of the dying, the feelings that are often present in the sickroom might become bearable. (p. 1730)

This is also true for psychotherapists, who have shared the client's life. How little we sit with death. How quickly we adjust to the news, and go on with our lives.

If we cannot sit with the dead person in the hospital room, the wake and funeral may provide some opportunity to reflect on the client's life as we experienced it, our feelings of loss, and the sharp edge between life and death. Attending funerals has been, for me, an opportunity for closure. The client whose funeral I attend does not just disappear over the weekend, but is said goodbye to. It settles me, and prepares me for the next person I sit with, including myself.

11
Caring for Ourselves

My supervisor tells this story: If your livelihood was dependent on a $125,000 tool, you would take good care of it. You'd clean it daily, and make sure it received routine maintenance. You'd safeguard it against abuse, protect it against overuse and breakage, and you'd lock it away at night.

Unfortunately, psychotherapists do not care as well for their most important tool, themselves.

Psychotherapy is a difficult enough profession. Its powers and difficulties lie in the two-way emotional bonds between client and therapist. Psychotherapy is enhanced by the gifts of empathy that enable practitioners to feel the client's pain and confusion, and the client to understand that his or her story is heard and appreciated. The empathic attachment to clients in pain guarantees that practitioners will also feel pain. Through the attachment to the client the therapist's heart aches with the client's.

At another level, quality practice also guarantees that the clinician will ache for herself or himself. The client's issues and expressions, heard and appreciated, will touch the practitioner's hidden emotions and confront unexplored fears and hurts. In psychotherapy, the clinician will often feel disquieted. Sometimes one cannot explain why he or she responded in a certain way, or used a particular tone of voice. These signals require gentle introspective inquiry. Although psychotherapy training suggests attentiveness to the client, too often therapists fail to be attentive to their own feelings.

As difficult as psychotherapy is, HIV-related work is more difficult, for many reasons. The most obvious reason is that the work may deal not only with psychopathology and maladjustment, but also with a chronic and life-threatening disease and its stresses, with concerns regarding a foreshortened life, and with the waxing and waning of hope. Another reason for its difficulty comes from the client's having a condition with sociopolitical implications. Both before and after HIV infection the client with an alternative lifestyle has been affected by and has reacted to the community. After infection, the HIV-positive client is affected also by medical, social, and political institutions that have insufficient resources and services. A psychotherapist doing case management that involves helping the client locate and obtain scarce services may become quickly frustrated with their unavailability—a feeling that parallels the client's frustration.

Furthermore, this work is complicated by continual evidence of personal vulnerability. But while the client is physically vulnerable, the therapist is reminded of both physical *and* professional vulnerabilities. Stressed by the personal meaning of facing a person with a life-threatening disease, the therapist is additionally stressed by the personal and professional meaning of being unable to rescue this client.

For many, the reflexive response to these feelings of vulnerability is the mounting of defenses. Some may choose to avoid HIV-positive clients altogether. Others may work with them but decide to toughen themselves, that is, become unfeeling, and distant. This may entail denial of pain and, consequently, a failure on the therapist's part to resolve these personal issues. Other practitioners may, over time, become "burned out," with onset of *chronic* feelings that may include anger, demoralization, dysphoria, subclinical depression, and feelings of being overwhelmed and powerless. In any case, the professional as well as the client suffers.

Work with HIV-positive persons is not necessarily accompanied by a defensive posture or the threat of burnout. Rather, it is unreflective psychotherapeutic work with HIV-positive persons and failures in self-care that can contribute to demoralization. Lack of introspection, which can be a product of avoiding supervision of psychotherapy for oneself, may result in an emphasis on psychotherapeutic product instead of process, on grandiose rescue fantasies, and lack of attentiveness to oneself. Unfortunately, because so many psychotherapists have the need to appear knowledgeable and in control, care of themselves is often more difficult than care of others. To others, a therapist can well explicate the possibilities in vulnerability for growth as well as pain but, feeling stressed or grandiose, may fail to accept those lessons for himself or herself. The phrase, "Take my advice, I'm not using it!" is all too often true.

This chapter, written at the conclusion of 2 and one-half years of full-time work at an inpatient and outpatient AIDS hospital, suggests several means to avoid AIDS-related burnout. In the first part, the therapist is urged to follow a course of coming to terms that parallels that of the client. The second and third parts suggest other strategies for this work, including the consideration of process as opposed to product as a criterion of success. The final section is written for those in institutional settings.

COMING TO TERMS

It is probably safe to say that many become therapists because they believe they can make a difference. Some feel that by helping others, they can change situations reminiscent of those they could not change as children; consequently, they can feel in control. Others may feel they have special talents, and should contribute time to those who have special needs. Others may believe their professional training enables them to make decisions for other people, to offer strong opinions that should be heeded.

Each of these motives contains, in one measure or another, a grandiosity that falls hard in the face of the chronic and life-threatening illness that is AIDS. As well, many HIV-positive clients, who have faced lifetimes of difficulties, also sorely test the good intentions of psychotherapists who measure their efficacy by client compliance.

Oftentimes the grandiosities—and their sharp contrasts with reality—are laughably obvious. On my office wall hangs a gold-sealed diploma and internship certificate and a state license, all in mahogany frames. So they are behind me when the client faces me and says, "My HIV test is positive, Doctor. But, I have to ask, why me?" And then the elegant documents and frames dissolve into their essential meaninglessness and there are just two persons with each other, facing the unanswerable.

A primary goal for the psychotherapist who works with HIV-positive clients, as much as for clients, is a coming to terms with professional and personal grandiosities and the unanswerables of mortality and fate. Only through this process can we reduce the several sources of stress that are inherent in this work. The primary source of stress is the existential: This work confronts us with the client's mortality and indeed, with our own. To deny the client's mortality is to do him or her a grave and significant disservice and would essentially be malpractice. The client's mortality, in the face of AIDS, underlies the psychotherapy. A similar danger dwells in the therapist's denial of his or her own mortality. If that denial continues, the therapist is effectively separated from his or her own deepest existential anxieties. Thus separated from his or her own humanity, this therapist then effectively separates from the client—"I am different; I am not mortal like the client"—precluding any meaningful therapeutic relationship.

One's helplessness in the face of inevitable death is foreshadowed by therapists' feelings of powerlessness with ill or noncompliant clients. The goal-driven therapist who wants to "make a difference" and who must see manifest proof of change can be continually thwarted by the client's illness, or by the client's inability to respect and gratify the clinician's grandiosity. If, in one's grandiosity, the therapist dares to enter a power struggle, death and its foreshadowings always win.

Rather than struggle with inevitabilities, the therapist should come to terms with them. Coming to terms, then, means the therapist's gradual introspective process of appreciating the limits of one's powers and, also, the gifts that one brings to the therapeutic relationship. It means, simplistically speaking, accepting the realities of life, that being alive means to be vulnerable, and to be vulnerable means to be open to pain as well as joy. Within the therapeutic relationship, which parallels other relationships, openness to the existential realities of the client and oneself means being open to the gift of the relationship as well as to the pain of inevitable loss.

Psychotherapy for the Therapist

The coming to terms requires an attentiveness to one's own feelings, and the understanding of them through our own psychotherapy. These feelings are important because we experience the client and ourselves through them. Yet, how often do we take the time and sit with our feelings when the client is with us, or after the session is over? Do we listen to our internal messages of fatigue, impotence, joy, hunger, rejection—including self-rejection—sadness, dread? If we do not listen, is the reason because we fear what we would find? Or is it because our tool is not so valuable, or has hardly any value?

The processing of these feelings and coming to terms with grandiosity and mortality, taking into account the idiosyncratic shadings of one's personal past and defenses, cannot normally be accomplished without professional assistance. It is even more unlikely when the issues are as potent as death. And even if it could, why should this journey be done in aloneness? One would not expect the HIV-positive client, or any client, to embark on a solitary journey of self-therapy. If a therapist is to work with HIV-positive clients, a course of psychotherapy is necessary to process his or her own deepest fears and fantasies, and to understand that the client's journey is, also, our own.

Supervision

In addition to one's own psychotherapy, supervision that focuses primarily on the therapist's emotional responses is necessary. To practice generally without supervision is dangerous enough. But to treat HIV-positive persons without assistance is to invite technical problems and countertransferential interference of the sort that leads one into incompetence.

The technical aspects of general practice are never static. In cognitive–behavioral work, new techniques or refinements as well as new scientific findings are continually emerging. One can never work competently or securely without access to professional seminars and journals. However, many would not attend continuing education conferences if state licensing bodies did not require it. And what should one read to stay abreast? New HIV-related information is available weekly, and the emotional lives of the clients change with it. A newspaper prematurely reports an experiment on one person; thousands respond with misguided optimism. Supervision by a master therapist who supports professional development and technical expertise can help one keep abreast.

Regarding supervision of the emotional aspects of this work, consider the supervisor/supervisee relationship as analogous to that of therapist/client. What one seeks from one's supervisor is exactly what the client must seek from the therapist: attentiveness, acceptance, regard, and direction.

PROCESS OVER PRODUCT

Therapists, as do other service providers, often measure success in concrete ways: the obtaining of services, achievement of therapy goals, reduced stress, among these. Facing institutional inertia and chronically unable to obtain needed services for a client, a social worker may quickly become frustrated and burn out. Physicians and nurses, facing patients who die despite their best efforts, become depressed. Psychotherapists, experiencing clients as noncompliant or unable to attain concretely stated psychotherapeutic goals, may decide to avoid HIV-positive clients. Everyone wants to feel efficacious, powerful, and in control—in sum, successful.

An example of product-oriented professional efforts are those that attempt to enforce compliance with medical directives. A request for a psychological consultation came from a physician who was unable to convince a woman to agree to a surgical procedure that would allow tube feeding. The woman, who had AIDS-related wasting syndrome, was becoming thinner. The physician said he felt that he had failed in his goal of convincing her to extend her life.

In this case, and with many others that involve the seemingly reasonable goals of caretakers—including physicians, family members, and therapists—clinicians become frustrated and, sometimes, angry because the client is being unreasonable and noncompliant. In the above case, the woman's refusal to have tube feedings despite her weakened condition seemed unreasonable. The physician's desired product: a reasonable decision to have surgery.

The consultation sought not to persuade the patient to have surgery but, rather, to suggest to the physician that he should consider a redefinition of "success." In this instance, the physician's success in his relationship with the patient was evidenced by respect for the woman's decision, and acceptance of her autonomy.

Therapists, too, have many similar issues regarding success. Too many measure themselves only by achievement of therapy goals, behavior changes, or interpretations that produce insight. These professionals respond with disappointment tinged with anger when a client seems disrespectful of or not compliant with the same goals. Several aspects are not considered, however. For one, reasonable goals, or products, may not seem reasonable or possible to persons who have endured an unreasonable life. Lifetime patterns are not easily altered, and perhaps never will change. Genuine differences of opinion regarding quality and quantity of life may be voiced. Similarly, some clients may become ill or experience cognitive dysfunction, precluding achievement of concrete goals. In so many ways beyond the therapist's control therapy goals may never be achieved.

If this is the case, should the therapist avoid these difficult cases or become discouraged if no changes are clearly evident? An alternative is a different measurement of success: The psychotherapeutic relationship. The practitioner should inquire of himself or herself if the best available consultative skills and knowledge was provided. Then, the therapist should ask, was the application of these skills joined by compassion and acceptance? In short, did the therapist provide the bases for a genuine relationship?

In subtle ways, the therapist touches every client. Perhaps few clients respond in the way that we would prefer. Perhaps some make decisions we would regard as wrong. But our gratification should come not from the client's behaviors that fulfill our needs, but in our conduct that regards the client's needs. The physician did not fail in his inability to persuade the patient to agree to surgery; rather he succeeded by compassionately accepting the patient's control over her own life. The psychotherapist's success is measured in the quality of the relationship.

OTHER STRATEGIES

Keep in Touch

Too often in regular practice, clients terminate and disappear. They may have been engaged in therapy, or they may have endured 5 sessions and then terminated. But the clinician is too busy to maintain any form of contact. In AIDS-related work, after a person leaves therapy, the fantasy that the person died may emerge. Ask clients who terminate to stay in touch with a simple message left on an answering machine, or a postcard now and then. Alternatively, make a brief phone call every couple months, just to convey the message of your concern. This keeps the person alive for the therapist, and reduces the sense of loss that can accumulate over time.

Memorialize Clients

For any therapist, either in private practice or in an institutional setting, there is a need to say goodbye to the client who has died. Those in institutional settings, such as hospitals, often face the "disappearance" of someone they have known but who died while they were not at work. Sometimes, depending on the clientele, there may not be a funeral or memorial service. We know that funerals are for the living; we should take advantage of them so we can say our goodbyes, and give ourselves closure.

Several staff members at an AIDS center in New York would, at the end of a weekly meeting, name those who had died recently. It gave everyone a few moments to recollect, and feel.

Weisman's Suggestions

Weisman (1981) gives three recommendations to alleviate caregivers' plight. The first he calls "least possible contribution" (p. 167). By this he means not doing as little as possible, "but doing only a little bit beyond the ordinary" (p. 167): an intervention that will make the biggest contribution with the least strain. His second suggestion is the sharing of critical incidents with colleagues: "Colleagues may have nothing more to offer than mutual concern and willing ears, but they can help us learn how to listen for echoes of disappointment and promises unkept" (p. 167). The final suggestion is that of a psychological autopsy or "absent witness" process in which the former patient (who has terminated or died) is asked to critique the professional's care. The absent witness is asked questions such as "What did you want that you did not get?" and "What should have been done that wasn't?" (p. 167). The technique is meant to be evaluative rather than critical, and can often help the caregiver more realistically assess the services provided.

Avoiding Excessive AIDS Work

The experience of AIDS moves many persons to become involved in many aspects: not only in psychotherapy but in fundraising, advocacy, and political lobbying. Sometimes, this involvement also stems from identification with those affected, hyper-responsibility, personal emphases on caretaking, and other personal reasons. The result, for some, is an "AIDS-related lifestyle," which has little content that is not AIDS. Work time involves AIDS; afterwork time involves AIDS and there is insignificant leisure time. Such a lifestyle can result in emotional erosion over time as one attempts to confront and control the various medical and sociopolitical processes. While AIDS asks much of society, individuals must also temper their zeal, and allow themselves the energy for the long run. One cannot ignore vacations, attention to healthy friends, aesthetic interests, recreation and hobbies, or one will not remain psychologically strong. The psychotherapist who has HIV-positive clients must judiciously decide how many are sufficient, and intersperse them with clients whose existential situations are less critical.

THERAPISTS IN INSTITUTIONAL SETTINGS

Some mental health professionals work in settings—such as hospitals, nursing homes, and social service agencies—that care for many HIV-positive clients. In such institutional work, the practitioner will experience a greater intensity of emotions regarding AIDS. This can be due to several reasons: Greater exposure to these clients, institutional and systemic problems of inertia and entropy, and the more-intense dedication that draws the practitioner to these settings. Persons in these settings must take special care to avoid emotional fatigue and demoralization.

In some settings, however, administrators are not attuned to the emotional aspects of continuous work with HIV-positive clients. Their primary concerns are scheduling, totals of client-contact hours, and paperwork. Others, however, are more enlightened, and realize the gift they can bring to employees by acknowledging their emotional needs.

The elements in the following sections should be considered.

Seeking Emotional Support

In a setting that is both professionally and emotionally taxing, professionals must be able to confide in and draw strength from one another. The confidences, ideally, should include discussion about personal pain and professional errors, as well as noncontroversial topics. Unfortunately, hierarchies and personalities sometimes prevent this. In a setting without a collegial atmosphere, clinicians may consider:

- Advocacy of a team approach, ideally within a nonhierarchical model.

In a larger facility, this may be suggested as a pilot project, perhaps in one part of the institution, such as on one hospital ward. Team members should be chosen on a basis of their personal comfort with each other, as well as their professional expertise. One stated goal of the team will be to provide professional and emotional support to each member.

- Seeking peer support inside or outside the institution.

This can be accomplished either by founding or joining a professional support or peer supervision group, or by hiring a supervisor who can provide professional support. Thus, one can join a group whose members belong not on the basis of rank or title, but on the basis of a shared interest in mutual support.

- Additional use of professional development techniques, such as retreats away from the workplace, to enable staff to reduce stress and form personal relationships.

Work "Mix"

Because of the stressful nature of the work, the number of direct client-contact hours will necessarily be lower than in other settings. Employees and administrators should encourage a mix of activities, that could include supervision and education, research, clinical publications, and attendance at professional meetings.

Administrators should consider a calendar of continuing education seminars and conferences that concern the emotional needs of staff as well as technical expertise. While you can bring a staff member to the fountain but not necessarily make him or her think, making these conferences mandatory will indicate administrators take these issues seriously. If institutions neglect staff members' morale and emotional factors, this may signal lack of concern about clients' well-being.

Clinicians should observe strict rules on overtime, even if their administrators do not. Institutions often reward quantity of work rather than quality of care. A fatigued clinician who habitually works overtime is neglectful of clients, as well as of him or herself.

Special Projects

Encouraging staff to participate in special projects and task forces is one means of letting staff know they are important. While administrators may have to concern themselves with crisis management, others should be encouraged to help the institution plan for the next decade, or to pursue solutions to specific problems. Two such projects suggested at a hospital were the creations of a multidisciplinary task force to plan for the special needs of female clients, as well as that of an ongoing continuing education program regarding the needs of IVDUs.

Special projects may include research and such activities as organization of a patient art show and videotaping of patient autobiographies (to be given to family members). Small intrainstitution grants may be made available to fund such activities.

Working Out "Sideshow" Disputes

Within an institution, staff members can avoid the anxiety that accompanies patient care by engaging in disputes. These internecine battles may seem, on the surface, to be rationally based and may involve such issues as turf, allegations of poor performance, and personality conflicts. Normally, such issues are resolved gracefully or, at least, the combatants attempt as professionals to avoid open disagreements. However, in some settings, these disputes continue interminably, or the furor is disproportionate to the manifest causes. When this occurs in an AIDS setting, participants should consider the possibility that these sideshows allow them to avoid patient contact and whatever negative feelings are evoked by that contact. It may be that instigation and continuation of high-pitched political and professional disputes serve to distract and entertain, allowing respite from anxieties and other difficult feelings evoked by daily work with very ill and difficult clients. The anxieties caused by the disputes are preferred, at some level, to those other feelings.

If a pattern of such disputes becomes evident, staff members could attempt to determine if contentiousness serves them by distracting them from other job-related anxieties.

CLAIMING THE GIFT

Despite the anxiety-provoking and otherwise difficult nature of this work, it nevertheless is about living and about confirming life. That is sometimes easily forgotten amidst the the fears, the evoked feelings, and the losses.

Perhaps the strongest statement that the psychotherapist, as well as the client, can make in the face of HIV infection is a renewed commitment to claim the gifts of growth and life. Faced with the inevitability of death, the therapist—through the relationship with the client, attentiveness to oneself, psychotherapy, and supervision—again becomes cognizant of the miracle of life. In our awe, we can find new meaning, new courage, and new realizations of how precious every moment can be. In celebrating the preciousness of life, we thrive.

PART 4

OTHER HIV-RELATED ISSUES

12

HIV Screening and Issues
of Early Detection

No topic is more emblematic or indicative of the changes in attitudes that have taken place in the late 1980s than that of HIV testing for persons who show no symptoms of HIV-related illnesses. Shilts (1988) well describes the absolute opposition to testing that until recently had permeated the gay AIDS movement. The stance was that since there were no medical interventions available to an HIV-positive but asymptomatic person, there was little point to knowing if one was positive.

In 1989, with announcements from the National Institutes of Health (NIH) that zidovudine used in asymptomatic individuals seemed to stave off opportunistic infections and prolong lives, organized opposition to testing began to change. In August, Gay Mens Health Crisis began to place newspaper advertisements with the headline, "If you haven't taken the antibody test for the AIDS virus, think about it." It continued, "Because if you test positive, you now have choices," including immune system tests, and prophylactic uses of zidovudine and aerosolized pentamidine. The *New York Times* featured the about-face on page one (Lambert, 1989), saying the organization "joined a growing nationwide shift among former critics of testing who agree that new drugs that fight AIDS can prolong life, particularly if the virus is detected early."

The newspaper advertisements and press conference pronouncements created a new influx of persons to be tested and, if positive, to be treated prophylactically. Unfortunately, the opportunities for preventive care were con-

147

fined, largely, to those with financial resources and the good fortune to live in urban areas that had savvy doctors attuned to AIDS.

The ideal situation for someone contemplating the HIV test is to have it conducted confidentially by a private physician knowledgeable about HIV, who will interpret positive results in the context of a person's overall physical condition and immediately begin prophylactic medication. Some argue that the individual should not seek insurance reimbursement, if available, for the tests and prophylactic medication, and should instead pay out of pocket and keep the HIV status secret from insurance companies. The downside of this stance is the eventual drain on a person's financial resources. Bunis (1989) described a man who spent thousands of dollars rather than life insurance claims, fearing his employer would learn of his condition. Self-paying patients, unfortunately, to conserve money may endanger their health by stinting on physicians' office visits, expensive testing procedures, and prophylactic medication, as well as on other aspects of improving well-being, including leisure activities and psychotherapy.

A potentially HIV-positive person with meager personal and financial resources, or dependent on public medical care, needs assistance to take a hard and sophisticated look at the decision to test.

One major question for a person without symptoms and considering HIV testing is whether prophylactic care is available. If the person has few resources, the availability of subsidized prophylactic medication and medical care must be considered. Furthermore, the client should be advised to be knowledgeable about the community's conditions of confidentially or anonymous testing. Confidential testing generally means the person's name is recorded along with the result. In some locales, names of HIV-positive persons are reported to health agencies; these agencies may now conduct or may be contemplating contact tracing: when someone is found to be HIV-positive, the sex or needle-sharing partners may be approached and told they have been exposed to HIV. Anonymous testing means no name is recorded and is usually conducted only with code numbers. An individual who is tested by a private physician or a public agency must inquire whether reporting to others occurs or is required.

These public health agencies are seldom integral parts of medical systems that would immediately provide medical care. Typically, a public-agency client who learns he or she is HIV-positive is counseled about what community resources are available, but then is left to his or her own resources to obtain aid. Then, depending on the community, unless acute symptoms exist, the client may have to wait weeks or months between testing and the first medical appointment.

Another difficulty clients face is finding a physician who will begin the prophylactic treatments immediately. The NIH studies of zidovudine in asymptomatic persons were reported in the press before they were published in scientific journals. As a result, some conservative physicians said they would wait until they could scrutinize the studies before initiating new treatment protocols. Now protocol results have been published (Volberding et al., 1990; Fischl et al., 1990), a NIAID conference has recommended zidovudine therapy for both symptomatic and asymptomatic persons with CD-4 counts less than 500 (NIAD, 1990), the FDA has approved the therapy for asymptomatic individuals, and physicians are being urged to start prophylaxis in persons with CD-4 counts below 500 (Friedland, 1990). Yet, even in this area there is no unanimity. The editors of the British medical journal *Lancet* (1990) are skeptical, and Phair et al. (1990) have suggested no prophylaxis for *pneumocystis pneumonia* be given to asymptomatic individuals until their CD-4 cells measure 200 or fewer.

Another related difficulty is the expense of prophylactic medications. Zidovudine initially cost the individual about $8,000 yearly but is now less expensive due to use of smaller dosages and the manufacturer's decision to reduce the price. Some infected persons do not have the financial resources to purchase prophylactic medication, and federal and other subsidies have been insufficient (Chase, 1989). In the United States, the costs of early intervention—that is, HIV treatment and PCP prophylaxis—could be $5 billion per year (Arno, Shenson, Siegal, Franks, & Lee, 1989). It is unclear whether federal or local governments are willing to fund this enterprise.

There are also hidden problems and costs. In some areas, prominently New York and San Francisco, networks lead resourceful persons to physicians who provide medications outside of recommended protocols. But others outside such networks may have to do expensive, time-consuming, and frustrating searching for knowledgeable physicians. Moreover, those who seek medications that either are not authorized for AIDS or not generally available will have to pay for them.

Therefore, urged to take the test, many persons may find themselves having to wait for clinic appointments, unable to pay for or have access to subsidized prophylactic treatments, and facing unknowledgeable physicians and other hidden problems.

Helping a person decide whether to take the HIV test, and enabling him or her to acknowledge and respond to the test results, has become a subspecialty with a growing number of training courses provided by private and governmental organizations. Some therapists in private practice may find themselves working with persons who, having engaged in high-risk activities, are debating whether to be tested so they can begin prophylactic treatments. Other clients may have to take the HIV test if they want life insurance or visas to enter certain countries. Whatever the reasons, the mental health practitioner should consider a two-part process: The first is a pretest assessment, to help the client determine if he or she indeed wants to have the test, and to assess if the client is emotionally able to take the test; the second is posttest counseling, which aids the client in acknowledging and responding to the results.

Therapist's Knowledge and Personal Stance

Because the decision to face a possible positive HIV result is so obviously crucial to a client's well-being, providing counseling without consideration of several issues would be tantamount to malpractice. These issues include assessing your own views on HIV testing and the extent of your knowledge of community resources for the HIV-positive person.

A Well-considered Stance on Testing

Some counselors believe that everyone who has had sex since 1979 or a transfusion before mid-1985 should be tested, unless there is a risk that a person testing positive will commit suicide or homicide in anger. Others, however, will dissuade persons from testing based on an appraisal of risk behaviors: these behaviors include sex with an individual likely to be infected, or needle-sharing. Those without risk behaviors or a small chance of infection are discouraged from testing, in the belief that taking the test is anxiety-provoking for anyone, and also because the fact of having taken the test, regardless of the outcome, can result in discrimination.

Because the counselor's stance affects the precounseling process, the therapist must determine his or her stance, be able to defend it, especially to himself or herself, and admit to the sociopolitical and emotional factors that determined that stance. While the counselor's position should not be imposed on the client, it is likely that this prejudgement "leaks" into the process. This is especially true if the decision is part of an ongoing therapeutic relationship during which you have communicated, subtly or not, your beliefs regarding testing.

HIV and Community Resources

Competent counseling requires knowledge not only about HIV transmission and other medical issues, but also about community resources. While many clients may have the personal resources to seek out information from such sources as private physicians and community groups, other less resourceful clients may rely solely on the HIV counseling. Even if the counselor is uncomfortable with the client's dependent stance, he or she should have information to judge if the client has the sufficient knowledge to make an informed decision regarding testing. If the therapist is comfortable providing a full spectrum of community information that will enable the client to make an informed decision, a great deal of knowledge is required.

PRETEST COUNSELING

The counselor needs to be active in the pretest counseling process. The responsibility includes not only helping a client make a decision regarding taking the test, but assessing the client's motivation, reflecting it back, and assessing whether the test will be emotionally harmful.

Some mental health professionals work in HIV screening clinics, providing quick assessments and counseling for persons about to take the HIV test. These individuals have a great deal of responsibility in performing a difficult task quickly. The following description of process may aid clinic counselors, as well as therapists who have an enduring relationship with the client.

The counselor, in a relationship with a person considering HIV testing, acts both as educator and consultant. The model for this process is that of a cost–benefit analysis with the consultant's professional advice. This advice can, of course, be rejected by the client.

The decision-making process should include the following five points.

1. Time Since Last Risk Behavior

A client should be advised about the 6-month window of nondetectability of the HIV antibody. A person may want to have a test anyway, to quell anxiety or to explore early intervention if the result is positive. But if the risk behavior occurred fewer than 6 months ago, a negative test result will not be conclusive. Another test should be recommended, as well as prevention counseling that urges an end to the risk behaviors.

2. Are There Physical Symptoms That Concern the Client?

If the client manifests physical symptoms, he or she may want to discuss them with a physician before taking the test. If the client has avoided that discussion, the counselor should learn why. If the discussion has occurred and the individual was told the symptoms are not HIV-related, the client's determination to take the test raises psychological issues.

3. What Are the Emotional/Motivational Aspects?

What is the motivation to take the test? Is it emotional (to relieve anxiety or depression); pragmatism ("My partner and I want to stop using condoms and so we want to make sure we're negative") or one of physical concern?

Have risk behaviors occurred? That is, has the client had sex with someone possibly bisexual, gay, or an intravenous drug user, or has he or she shared needles, or had a transfusion before mid-1985? It is also possible that the chance of transmission is highly unlikely and the stated emotional motivation may have another source that requires exploration (see Chapter 15).

Does the client know of sex or needle-sharing partners who are ill? If former partners are ill or have died, this may indicate a greater chance of testing positive.

Is the client pregnant or is there a likelihood of pregnancy in the future? Does the woman want to be tested before becoming pregnant or is she already pregnant? If the woman is already pregnant, are there specialty services such as counseling centers and prenatal clinics for HIV-positive persons available in the community for referrals? If not, is the counselor part of an integrated service delivery system that will provide care for the pregnant HIV-positive woman and, possibly, a baby?

4. Costs Versus Benefits

What is the client's prediction of his or her emotional response to the test? Does the client make a clear denial of suicidal intent?

What is the therapist's assessment of the likely emotional response to the test result? What is your best assessment of the possibility of negative emotional impact, depression, feelings of revenge, anxiety, and, of course, suicide? Does the client have the emotional resources to deal with a positive result? Is there current depression or preexisting psychiatric illness that can be exacerbated? Some statement of your assessment should be shared with the client. If the client rejects your advice, how will this affect the therapeutic relationship?

The patient's level of knowledge, when the discussion regarding testing is begun, may be an indicator of his or her emotional and cognitive resources. Does the client prefer to remain oblivious to the ramifications of a positive result?

What are the likely pragmatic costs to the client, including discrimination in the workplace, life and medical insurance, or housing? If an employer learns of the positive result, can termination occur? Even if the termination is a violation of law, a lengthy legal process can ensue. Is a positive result likely to jeopardize insurance benefits? Is the client's housing situation stable?

Is continued drug use involved? How will this be affected by a positive or negative result? Is the client willing to enter a drug treatment program now?

Will sexual behavior change? Is the person currently using safer sex? Will sexual behavior change if there is knowledge of positivity?

Will a testing result provide motivation to improve lifestyle, health?

Will a negative result end anxiety? If not, then other psychological issues should be explored.

5. Supportive Resources Available if HIV-Positive

If there is a positive result, does the client have immediate access to HIV-knowledgeable physicians who can explain the result in the context of available medical knowledge and the client's physical condition? Can prophylactic medication be started if indicated?

Is public medical treatment, including prophylactic medication, available?

Can the patient tolerate the waiting time between a positive result and available medical care?

If there are no knowledgeable persons nearby, does the patient have the resources and ability to travel?

Does the patient have resources, or is funding available, to pay for medical care, including prophylactic treatment?

Does the patient have access to research protocols?

Will family members, friends, and/or a lover be supportive if the client is HIV-positive? Will there be negative ramifications? Will the client reveal a positive test result to these persons?

OTHER REASONS FOR TESTING

Insurance

Persons who apply for life insurance and some medical insurance policies may be required to take HIV tests. These tests are often conducted by nursing and laboratory services paid by the insurance company. A person who may have some risk behaviors and seeks insurance may be advised to be tested anonymously before applying for insurance. If the anonymous test is negative, then the insurance test is very likely to be negative. But applying and then withdrawing an insurance application, or being tested and found positive, may have negative implications.

Foreign Travel

The State Department's Citizens Emergency Center has compiled a list of countries that require documentation of a negative HIV test from some or all travelers. Most require the test only if there is a longterm stay or work involved but some countries do not accept tests conducted in the United States (see Wade, 1990). Because these rules change, contact the State Department or the country's embassy before travel.

POSTTEST COUNSELING

Neither a positive nor a negative result indicates the end of the professional's responsibility to the client.

In the case of a positive result, the responsibilities are great and are dictated by the professional's relationship to the client. A counselor in a screening clinic must assess emotional and other effects of the positive result, and make appropriate referrals. A psychotherapist in an ongoing relationship must assess the client's situation and reconsider the therapeutic contract. Both the client and the therapist must reassess goals and needs, and the therapist must decide whether he or she can provide what is needed. The new therapeutic contract should enable the client to attain the stated goals and improve quality of life (see Chapter 5).

A negative result is a happy occurrence, but also requires a professional response that includes:

1. Assessment to determine if the client has an appropriate response to the result. If a client's worry or dysphoria does not diminish after a negative result, new hypotheses need to be considered: Did the client understand the result? Have there been ongoing, undisclosed risk behaviors? Is there a preexisting psychopathology, such as a delusional disorder?
2. Prevention counseling, tailored to the client's needs. A client who is likely to continue needle sharing needs to be educated about the use of bleach to clean needles. Those who have feared AIDS due to risky sex behaviors need information about safer sex practices including use of condoms, ejaculation outside the body, avoidance of drugs or alcohol when sex might be at issue, and assertiveness training to avoid pressures to engage in unsafe sex. This are described in more detail in the following chapter.
3. An emotional and existential assessment of the testing experience, followed by an evaluation of one's values and lifestyle. Many persons who feared a positive result find that a negative result provides them a new lease on life. They are able to refocus on old goals, set new meaningful goals, and discard some concerns that they now view as trivial.

13
Prevention Counseling

For practitioners and for organizations alike, a crucial HIV-related task of the 1990s will be prevention of HIV infection.

Unfortunately, prevention efforts continue to be hampered by lack of adequate evaluation of effectiveness. Even the assumptions upon which we have based prevention efforts have, over time, required evaluation and reconsideration. Moreover, prevention efforts are hampered by sociopolitical and cultural differences in communities, which may require narrowly focused efforts, as opposed to broad city-wide plans. In the case of work with IVDUs, especially, the cultural differences between those who would initiate prevention programs and their targets have led to missteps and oversights.

Many myths exist regarding AIDS prevention. As expressed and responded to by the Citizens Commission on AIDS for New York City and Northern New Jersey (1989), they include:

- Continued public AIDS education is no longer necessary because persons know about HIV. The response: ". . . large numbers of people still believe they can catch AIDS from drinking glasses, toilet seats and casual contact" (p. 2).
- Public service announcements have saturated us with AIDS information. Response: They have had limited impact because of infrequent and erratic airings.
- AIDS education for heterosexuals is not necessary. Response: AIDS spreads through heterosexual sex. The percentage of women and adolescents infected heterosexually is increasing.
- Adolescents do not need education additional to that provided in the schools. Response: "AIDS education that is limited to the classroom cannot

have the same impact as AIDS education that is repeated in many different settings" (p. 3).

The commission's responses and conclusions are to the point: Prevention efforts are sorely needed. Mental health specialists must be in the forefront of these efforts.

This chapter will first review the issues of prevention efforts, and will conclude with suggestions for the private practitioner.

EVALUATION

In 1987, Coates et al. published an agenda for AIDS-related psychosocial research that noted that although the need for careful evaluation of the effectiveness of AIDS prevention had already been identified, "little work which addresses this concern has been reported in the literature" (p. 26). Several years later, while some progress has been made, especially with gay men, evaluation of our prevention efforts is largely lacking. One reason, familiar to those who are primarily clinicians, is the great gap between research and practice that exists in many nonuniversity institutions. Clinicians, especially in medical settings, are extraordinarily pressed and have little time to conduct research that involves carefully controlled evaluation. Too often, institutions see this type of work as an expensive and time-consuming frill that diverts staff workers from clinical contact. Further, the world of research has become increasingly technical. A successful grant application is now a time-consuming process that requires an agency's investment in seed money and personnel time; research design, statistical and grantsmanship expertise; and contacts in a large number of granting agencies. Federal agencies, moreover, request highly specialized grant proposals. Some of these agencies will provide grants for only portions of a prevention project—either the evaluation (such as the Agency for Health Care Policy and Research) or only the actual prevention work and not the evaluation. This further complicates the grants process. While it is likely that clinicians who work with HIV-positive persons have many brilliant ideas for prevention, these never are tested because of the intricacies and problems of doing research.

Prevention efforts have also been hampered by the cultural differences between clinicians and their clients. This has been most noted in work with IVDUs. With these clients, prevention efforts have largely taken the form of programs that explain HIV transmission through dirty needles, and the importance of using clean needles, either by cleaning "works" with bleach or by participating in needle exchanges, where available. New observations of how IVDUs actually use and clean their drug-injection apparatuses found that "clean works" prevention efforts were inadequate (Kolata, 1989). Observers found, for instance, that water used to clean works was also used to liquefy drugs for injection. The possibly HIV-contaminated water, then, was also injected. Other shared devices, such as "cookers" in which drugs are mixed, and the cotton used for filters are also now being studied to determine if they are involved in HIV-infection. Prevention programs have to accomodate quickly to new findings.

SOCIOPOLITICAL CONSIDERATIONS

Development of large-scale or community-wide programs is significantly hampered by the volatile interaction between the sociopolitical composition of the community and the mortality and morality aspects of HIV. Early in the epidemic, many television station managers believed that their listeners would not tolerate condom advertisements, and kept them off the air. The Roman Catholic bishops of the United States, after years of public and private disagreement, finally decided that chastity was the only prevention method they could endorse. In New York City, black churches joined others in opposing needle exchange programs for active drug users, and the city's new mayor closed down the small pilot program in 1990.

Broad-spectrum community HIV prevention programs, which necessarily require broad backing, seem inevitably mired by efforts to create a message that is palatable to all in the community. Smaller, more narrowly focused programs, especially those not so dependent on public monies, may have more freedom to maneuver. Thus far, the best example of success with HIV prevention is the response of the homosexual community to the threat of AIDS. Prevention research with gay men has been plentiful, relative to other groups, and successful. Stall, Coates, and Hoff (1988) review some 24 studies regarding anal intercourse among gay men and find "dramatic behavior changes" (p. 878). One study they cite (Doll et al., 1987) found the rate of unprotected receptive anal intercourse was 27 times higher in 1978 than 1985. Much continuing seroconversion is attributed to loss of judgment due to use of alcohol or drugs, other studies they cite suggest (Stall, Wiley, McKusick, Coates, & Ostrow, 1986; Communication Technologies, 1987; see Martin, 1990). Linn et al. (1989) in a study of gay and bisexual men, found that those who had unsafe sex were more likely to be younger, of lower socioeconomic status, and minority group members, particularly Hispanic. Further, they had more sexual partners, engaged in sex more often, felt less in control of their sexual behavior, were unlikely to talk with partners about safe sex, and used recreational drugs more frequently.

Prevention success with gay men may be due to the features of urban gay life, where men openly identify themselves as gay and live in tightly knit, self-protective, politically active, and affluent communities where residents are not squeamish about discussing the realities of HIV prevention. The messages were narrowly focused to appeal to gay men, and did not face censorship by others. Unfortunately, what we have learned by research with these groups cannot necessarily be generalized to other groups. Stall, Coates, and Hoff (1988) noted that care should be taken about generalizing these data to men who engage in homosexual behavior who may be minority group members, not openly gay, or living in other settings.

One lesson for professionals focusing on group prevention strategies may be that large, heterogeneous groups are ill-suited for HIV prevention strategies. Rather, prevention programs may require identification of homogeneous, and smaller, subgroups. The prevention messages, then, can be sociopolitically focused and "narrow-cast" to specific groups, which may avoid community approbation.

One example of prevention activities that may have sociopolitical pitfalls is work with teenagers. A prevention specialist has choices about subgroups, settings in which to narrow-cast, and the message. If one were to target sexually active adolescents between 16 and 19, what approaches might be useful? While it may be that these persons can be approached in school, this may require a politic crafting of the message to parents' approval. A better program may be to target high school dropouts by way of street corner work, or to provide "commercials" at local musical activities. A joint concern for sexually active teenagers is adequate medical care, and perhaps a conjoint effort can be made between medical caregivers and AIDS prevention efforts.

PREVENTION LITERATURE

Psychotherapists should be familiar with the literature of prevention and behavior change, especially that related to health activities. The literature includes descriptions of both communitywide efforts and prevention efforts in the clinic and private practice settings. Work with smoking, seat belt use, and cholesterol levels, for example, has provided some insights into means of behavior change. Also, work with other groups may be adapted to HIV-prevention programs. For example, Marlatt and Gordon (1985) have made a valuable contribution with their work on relapse prevention. Other pertinent literature includes that on theoretical models of behavior change. Using elements of social learning theory (Bandura, 1977), communication/persuasion (Green, Reuter, Deeds, & Partridge, 1980), and the health belief model (Ajzen & Fishbein, 1980), Coates and Greenblatt (1990) have created an AIDS Risk Reduction Model. This is based on the premise that

> to avoid disease, people engaging in high risk activities first must perceive that their sexual behavior places them at risk for HIV infection and related morbidity and mortality. . . . [Then] individuals must be willing to commit themselves to changing their behavior. (pp. 1075–1076)

Other steps include provision of skills that would enable persons to change, and identification of those in the client's system who will support change.

Coates and Greenblatt (1990) wrote, "In its simplest formulation, behavior change requires information, motivation, skills, and an environment which supports healthful behaviors" (p. 1075).

In their 1988 article Kelly and St. Lawrence noted that effective health messages

> explicitly convey that: (a) the potential health threat from engaging in certain risk behaviors is great; (b) the individual who engages in these activities is personally vulnerable; (c) behavioral change can successfully reduce risk, and (d) the benefits from making risk behavior change are greater than the costs of failing to change. . . . [these messages] are most effective when they provide specific prescriptive advice on how to implement changes, explain the rationale for the recommended changes, and are encouraging in their tone. (p. 263)

PROGRAM TYPES

Thus far, AIDS-related prevention efforts have fallen generally into several categories of messages and means. These are:

- The widely disseminated "just say no"-type exhortations that translate into, "just stop it." With appetitive behaviors, sexual or drug-taking, skepticism is likely the realistic view of the efficacy of this approach.
- Street-type programs that provide prevention tools, such as condoms, clean needles or bleach, but without formal continuing relationships or follow-up; or street programs in which exaddicts act as AIDS educators without providing means (McAuliffe et al., 1987) or outreach workers to distribute vouchers for free detoxification treatment (Jackson & Rotkiewicz, 1987).
- Efforts that involve complex psychoeducation training, sometimes in the context of research attempts to determine efficacy.

The psychoeducational approach may include instruction on use of condoms, eroticization of safer-sex play, attitude change and assertive training, and cautions regarding the disinhibiting effects of alcohol and drugs. Unfortunately, much of the published literature concerns sexual behaviors of gay men, and its generalizability to other groups, including IVDUs, is doubtful. Research indicates some IVDUs engage in safer behaviors (Des Jarlais et al., 1989) and several programs have reported positive results with IVDUs and inmates (CDC, 1989). The private practitioner can find useful elements in these psychoeducational efforts.

One prevention project that focused on gay men resulted in an intervention manual which can be applied to private practice. Researchers intervened with gay men who had a history of high-risk behavior (Kelly, St. Lawrence, Hood, & Brasfield, 1989). Their interventions included AIDS risk education, behavioral self-management, assertiveness training, and relationship skills and social support development.

The educational component included information on HIV, infection, and it conceptualized behaviors on a continuum from high to less to lowest risk. Behavioral self-management training including having clients think of antecedents to their high risk behaviors, including drug or alcohol use and going to settings known for casual sex encounters. Leaders suggested strategies to lessen risk, as well as to generate and practice self-statements that emphasized safer sex practice. Assertiveness training included advance discussion with a potential partner of commitment to safe sex practice, refusals of pressures to have unsafe sex, and postponement of sexual involvement with someone one might want to get to know socially. The relationship skills and social support part included discussion of development of steady relationships with shared commitments to health. This training resulted in reduced frequency of high-risk practices and increased behavioral skills for refusing sexual coercion, with change maintained at an 8-month followup.

The noncopyrighted manual (Kelly & St. Lawrence, 1990) based on this work is available from Kelly at the Department of Psychiatry and Mental Health Sciences, Medical College of Wisconsin, 8701 Watertown Plank Rd., Milwaukee, WI 53226.

Des Jarlais and Friedman's (1988) review of studies of AIDS risk-reduction programs among IVDUs derived three principles for effective reduction:

1. "Basic information about AIDS and the transmission of HIV is needed . . . to generate motivation for risk reduction" (p. 869).
2. Information alone is insufficient, "the ready availability of means for behavior change is also critical" (p. 869). The corollary of this principle, the authors say, is that "providing means for reducing drug injection and providing means for 'safer injection' are complementary" (p. 869).
3. They offered this point with tentativeness due to limited data; it is based on behavior theory and knowledge about relapse: Sustained reinforcement for risk reduction behaviors must be available. This reinforcement can include the cognitive reinforcement of reduced fear, new social norms, and positive peer relationships, Des Jarlais and Friedman wrote.

Prevention among African-American and Hispanic men has been addressed by Peterson and Marin (1988). For minority gay men and IVDUs, they suggest more culturally sensitive channels of information (e.g., bilingual messages, radio instead of newspaper, use of friends and relatives). For drug-related community programs, they suggest more minority staff "who would be more accepted by minority addicts because of their knowledge of the minority culture values, particularly the social scripts related to respect and positive social relations" (p. 874). Others have written about prevention concerns specific to African-American and Hispanic women (Mays & Cochran, 1988) and children and adolescents (Brooks-Gunn, Boyer, & Hein, 1988; Flora & Thoresen, 1988).

PRIVATE PRACTITIONER STRATEGIES

In the 1990s, the individual psychotherapist must convey an HIV prevention message to all sexually active clients. For those engaging in risk behaviors, the message must be compelling, must be specific to the client's lifestyle, and must provide information, a rationale, and doable alternative behaviors. In the therapy office, and even in clinics and public health settings, the therapist may be freer to recommend a variety of prevention strategies tailored for the specific client than can the prevention expert working in a larger and more public setting.

HIV prevention should be presented as a means to the client's lifetime goals of health, good functioning, and social goals rather than as extrinsically required rules or regulations that intrude into a lifestyle. The beginning of the prevention conversation could be a discussion of those life goals. Most clients will readily say they want to be healthy and live a long life. Many want to procreate and see the children grow. Most want social support, from groups or from significant individuals. Given these goals, HIV prevention should be understood as means to attain these goals.

With this understanding, research and other programs suggests an AIDS prevention "menu" that includes information, attitude change, behavioral training, and social support.

Information

- Culturally aware and language-sensitive education about HIV, means of transmission, and other medical aspects.

This should be tailored to the client's needs and education level. Women, for example, should be told about the risks of heterosexual transmission and in utero transmission, especially if pregnancy is possible. IVDUs must obtain information both on transmission through needle sharing and sexual transmission. It is insufficient to hand pamphlets to clients. The information should be provided in a teaching context in which the clinician can answer questions, respond to puzzled looks and signs of embarrassment and other discomfort, and ask the client to feedback information learned. Brochures should be provided to reinforce and underline the information. Bilingual information should be available.

- Prevention information.

This includes specific information about safer sex, the use of condoms, clean needles, and discontinuation of sharing any devices involved in shooting up, including needle and syringe, cooker, filter, and water used for cleaning.

Kelly and St. Lawrence (1990), categorize activities into high, moderate and low risk. Anal sex, for example, believed to cause more membrane breakage and therefore provide more access to the receptive partner's blood system, is listed as high risk and should be discouraged. The researchers respond to questions and review such myths as "showering before sex (or after sex) is sufficient to reduce risk" (p. 34).

Use of latex condoms, preferably with nonoxynol 9, is advocated by prevention experts as a means to "safer sex." Clients should never use petroleum-based lubricants—such as Vaseline—which may damage latex, but should use K-Y jelly instead.

A demonstration of condom use on a penis-like object may be in order. The condom should be placed rolled up on the tip. A small reservoir should be allowed for semen, and then the condom should be unrolled along the penis. Also included in the demonstration should be instructions on how to remove the condom without fluid leakage. The proper technique is to hold the condom firmly on the penis, disengage from the partner, and remove the condom, continuing to hold the opening to avoid leakage.

Women who have sex with women are urged to protect themselves in various ways: With oral sex, to avoid exchange of vaginal secretions or blood the women should use a latex square known as a dental dam between mouth and the vaginal area. Some persons have cut and used condoms, which are thinner, as barriers. Partners who use objects such as dildos and vibrators should either use different ones for each person or sheath them with condoms and change the condoms before sharing. The objects should be cleaned well between uses.

For those with IVDU histories, the best protection is no injection. Assessment regarding motivation to end intravenous drug use and/or begin a drug treatment program should be done, with referrals made. But if the client is likely to continue injection, the danger of sharing needles and other works must be stressed. All parts of the drug-use paraphenalia, including the container used to "cook" the drugs, should be cleaned. If rubbing (ethyl) alcohol is available, it should be put into a glass and several times pulled up through the needle into the syringe, shaking well each time. Then, the works should be taken apart and, together with all other paraphenalia, soaked in the alcohol about 15 minutes. They should be left to dry. (Adopted from New York City Department of Health, 1987.)

If bleach (Clorox, for instance) is available, the client should follow these instructions: Mix one part bleach to ten parts water in a clean glass. Rinse the works with faucet water. Then draw up the bleach mix into the works or dropper, shake well; do this several times. Soak the unassembled works 15 minutes in the bleach solution, along with other equipment such as spoons or cookers. Rinse with clean water and let dry.

Oftentimes, however, water and filters employed in drug use can be contaminated, and clients must be warned against sharing these. Sometimes water is not available in "shooting galleries" and is shared by many users and thus contaminated. Also, cotton or cloth is used by many as filters, and can be contaminated. Filters and water cannot be shared without risk of contamination by HIV.

Work with IVDUs also should include discussion of sexual behavior, be the client gay or heterosexual. Heterosexual transmission is a great risk with this group, and they should receive prevention information regarding condoms.

Attitude Change

Based on the work of Kelly and St. Lawrence (1990; Kelly, St. Lawrence, Hood, & Brasfield, 1989), and that conducted by others, the following interventions could be attempted:

- Investigation and challenging of attitudes that link homosexuality with promiscuity and that place a high value on sexual expression with participation in high-risk sex.
- Eroticization of safer sex.

This includes notions that mutual masturbation and ejaculation outside the body can be as pleasurable as more traditional methods. This includes encouragement of additional conversation between partners about their physical and emotional sensations during sexual encounters. Partners are encouraged to talk more to each other about how they can better "pleasure" each other. Also suggested is use of more creative foreplay and different venues for sex. These include "talking dirty," more fantasy play, additional erotic touching, use of locations such as showers, disinhibition about ejaculation outside the body, such as on the partner's body—away from eyes and orifices and provided there are no cuts or scratches—as well as being ejaculated on.

Behavioral Training

The following behavioral techniques should be employed with the client:

- The client should be asked to analyze experiences in terms of "antecedents" or "trigger situations," that is, any facets of a situation that have led to risk-taking behaviors.

These antecedents may include specific persons or places, moods that preceded or accompanied the risky behavior, the quality of the risky encounters (hurried, casual, etc.), failure to consider actions, or use of disinhibiting substances, to name a few possibilities. The client should be asked to list and discuss these factors in detail.

- Planning of strategies to avoid dangerous antecedents or, as a secondary strategy, to change responses to them.

These strategies require a client to be willing to short-circuit or terminate an automatic, and likely complicated, stimulus–response sequence. Awareness of the sequence is insufficient. One must also have alternative behaviors, planned in advance. The client must have an awareness of new options and the skills to carry them through.

- Skills training, including assertiveness training, new cognitive strategies, and new behaviors.

They must be "in place" before the person encounters a possible risky situation. The therapist may consider assertiveness training, role playing, imaginal role playing, and the writing of scripts of dangerous situations with avoidance strategies and alternative behaviors as options.

- Cognitive modification of "self-talk" and self-reinforcement patterns, such as the notion, "frequent sex means I'm desirable."
- Reporting back to the therapist of the efficacy of the new skills, and the failures. The therapist should help the client analyze the problems, and allow for new strategies.
- Relapse prevention strategies, which include fantasizing about situations where unsafe behaviors may be provoked, and thinking through of prevention strategies that respond to these temptations.

Social Support

To plan and maintain behavioral changes, social support is required. This should include:

- Continuing therapist reinforcement for healthy behaviors.
- Encouragement of clients to seek social contacts who support risk reduction.

This includes encouragement of relationships in which sexual partners are committed to their mutual health, and participation in groups that provide supportive social norms for behavior change. For those with a history of intravenous drug use, such groups may include support groups or IV-focused Narcotics Anonymous groups.

Although prevention education has reduced the rates of seroconversions in the much-studied gay urban communities, by 1990 there was disturbing evidence of complacency. In Canada, researchers found 1988's seroconversion rate in a cohort of Canadian men to have increased over that of the previous year (Sestak et al., 1989). In Los Angeles, researchers found that 64% of 823 gay or bisexual men indicated they had engaged in at least one unsafe sexual

behavior during the previous 2 months. Only 9% of the men said they practiced safer sex always (Linn et al., 1989).

Individual's complacency, too, must be avoided. Some practitioners give
regular safer sex reminders to sexually active men and women. Others keep
pamphlets and other information in waiting rooms.

The task of prevention is two-fold: introduction of information in a useful
and understandable way that enables the client to understand that it is to be
part of a lifestyle, and reinforcement that obviates complacency. Mental health
organizations and private practitioners, because of their relationships with
clients that can last years, can make a unique contribution to prevention.

14

The Intravenous Drug User

One of the most mysterious and troubling aspects of human behavior is drug use, particularly intravenous drug use. And for many therapists, the most puzzling and unnerving client is the drug user. The use of a needle to inject drugs is, to many, distasteful and revolting. The criminality that fuels or is fueled by drug use provokes outrage, especially if one has been a crime victim. Many would regard IV drug users (also called injectors) as not members of society at all but rather as outsiders who have chosen to reject mainstream values in their pursuit of mood-altering chemicals. This outlook, however, is a classist one that ignores the ubiquitous nature of drug use across all class and race lines, and one that ignores the issue of how societies fail to provide hope in certain communities.

AIDS focuses attention on drug use for several reasons. The most obvious reason is that HIV is transmitted by needle sharing. One bodily fluid that serves as a medium for HIV transmission is blood. When drugs are injected, a small amount of blood is left in the needle or syringe. The syringe may then be passed to another user who, without adequate cleaning, uses it to inject. A small amount of the first user's blood intermingles with the the second user's heroin or other drug; this mix is injected into the second user. If there is HIV in the blood, that travels along into the second user. Currently, when one disentangles the CDC methods for reporting AIDS cases, we find that drug abusers now account for 25% of the cases, and the proportion is growing (Batki, Sorensen, Faltz, & Madover, 1988). In the northeastern United States, that proportion is much higher.

Another drug-related HIV issue is that of heterosexual transmission. A significant percentage of women infected through heterosexual transmission have partners who were infected through IV drug use. One study found the only predictor of HIV infection for former drug users who stopped injecting early in the AIDS epidemic (before 1982) was a history of sex partners who used intravenous drugs (Schoenbaum et al., 1989). HIV was found in 22 of 77 former drug users (28.6%) who reported one or more IVDU sex partners, compared with 13 of 82 (15.9%) who reported no IVDU sex partners. Another heterosexual drug-related risk is that offspring of couples in which the mother is HIV-positive may likewise contract HIV.

A less obvious relationship of drug use to AIDS is an indirect one: its effect on sexual behavior. Although the rock form of cocaine (crack) is smoked, not injected, substance stimulates sexual activity among participants who may fail to guard against infection from sexually transmitted diseases, including HIV (Kerr, 1989). The spread of STDs, such as syphilis, also may indirectly contribute to the spread of AIDS. In Africa, statistics indicate that female-to-male transmission is facilitated by concurrent genital ulcer disease in the male. A study of African-American adolescent crack users found that, for girls, a history of selling crack and the number of drugs used on a daily basis were associated with the number of reported risk behaviors for STD and HIV (Fullilove, Fullilove, Bowser, & Gross, 1990). These risk behaviors included failure to use a condom, prostitution for drugs or money, and combining sex with drug use. For boys, the number of drugs used on a daily basis and the description "I usually don't know ahead of time if I'm going to have sex— it just happens" predicted their number of risk behaviors.

Moreover, some believe that crack addiction encourages prostitution, which may facilitate HIV infection. Others (Day, 1988; Padian, 1988) doubt that prostitutes are responsible for further heterosexual HIV transmission.

Yet another less-obvious relationship of drugs to sex and AIDS are the effects of drug use on decision-making. Seroconversion has dropped significantly among the gay community in New York, due to education about safer sex. But many believe that the educational messages are disregarded when a person's judgment is impaired by use of substances such as cocaine or alcohol (Martin, 1990). An alternative explanation for the findings that drug use is associated with unsafe sexual practices (Linn et al., 1989) is that those who use recreational drugs are irresponsible about their health in many ways. Further, psychopathology, such as antisocial personality, may be involved (Ross, Glaser, & Germanson, 1988).

POLYSUBSTANCE ABUSE

Substance use more and more appears to be polysubstance use, at least in the large urban centers. About 74% of 377 subjects recruited from a methadone maintenance program, who said they had injected drugs since 1978, reported injection of cocaine (Schoenbaum et al., 1989). Heroin injectors not in treatment programs may also inject cocaine or a combination of cocaine and heroin, called speedball. Persons on methadone, which blocks the heroin high, may continue to use heroin and other opiates, cocaine, alcohol (Shikles, 1989) or speedball.

Methadone treatment programs sometimes are unable to respond effectively to urine test results that are positive for cocaine, and continue the methadone therapy. Those on methadone programs and others have ready street access to the substance: A Drug Enforcement Agency investigation found that there were street sales of methadone in New York City (Haislip, 1989). Further complicating the picture are new entries in the street drug markets, including a smokeable combination of cocaine (for the quick and short-lived high) and heroin (for an hours-long tranquilizing effect), and smokeable methamphetamine, called "ice."

Substance abuse counselors realize that the addictions are not only to the substances, but to a lifestyle of hustling, stealing, danger, and other "action."

PUBLIC DEBATE

The public debate regarding how to deal effectively with drugs is remarkable for its extremes. The U.S. governmental response to the drug crisis has been a call for increased enforcement. Increased enforcement means, to various persons, military involvement, new and larger prisons, military-style camps for drug sellers and users, and stricter punishment for those possessing an illegal substance. On the other side are those who argue that the drug war is "patently false, and the hope for victory so obviously futile" (Lapham, 1989, p. 44). Those who dare to speak about decriminalization of drugs usually provoke heated debate (Corcoran, 1989).

Much less attention—some would say none—has been paid to the biological, psychological, sociological, and political aspects of addiction, prevention, and treatment. In *Harpers,* Lapham (1989) wrote:

> To the extent that the slums can be seen as the locus of the nation's wickedness . . . , the crimes allied with the drug traffic can be classified as somebody else's moral problem rather than one's own social or political problem. (p. 47)

Apparent in some parts of society is a cynical and bitter stance regarding drug users. Add HIV infection and these persons often are society's throwaways. The cynical and bitter say quietly, "Let them die; they were useless—and worse—anyway."

Many mental health professionals, representative of a cross section of society, share these views. Hardened views regarding drug users require clinicians to recuse themselves from working with this population, to spare them yet more hostility. However, mental health practitioners, already inclined to understand the problems of others, have access to supervision and training that would enable them to understand the sources of substance abuse and the prejudices that affect drug users.

One useful tool to assess one's attitude regarding substance abuse is a scorable questionnaire contained in *AIDS and Substance Abuse* (Faltz & Rinaldi, 1988). Among the statements offered for response is, "You can only help a person with a drug problem if that person initiates a request for treatment." Faltz and Rinaldi (1988) emphasize that training in aspects of chemical dependency helps erode misconceptions that feed negative feelings about drug users.

Issues around treatment of drug users with HIV infection include stereotypical attitudes regarding drug users, psychotherapy treatment goals, assessment of the client's and therapist's abilities to achieve them, the availabilities of drug treatment programs and alternatives, and therapist's issues.

STEREOTYPES VERSUS REALITY

Among the most scorned of our citizens, intravenous drug users are seen as monolithic: psychopathic and criminal; severely disordered if not schizophrenic; of low intelligence, inarticulate, and unattractive. Disgust is not too strong a word to describe the public's reaction.

Some IVDUs share some or many of these attributes. Some are criminals, some are severely disordered, and some are of low intelligence. However, this does not describe all IVDUs, and likely not the majority. They include musicians, white collar administrators, and middle class housewives. Perhaps public attitude toward drug abuse differs depending on the social class of the user. When a concert violinist was arrested and charged with possession of cocaine and heroin, his attorney defended him by saying, "He is ill" and should enter a drug program (Gold, 1989). Later, this man, the first American to win the top prize in the Tchaikovsky violin competition in Moscow, was called "a casualty of the cruelly competitive world of classical music" (Hoban, 1989, p. 102). Few poor, African-American or Hispanic drug users are regarded as casualties of the cruel world of the slums.

Mikey is a 34-year-old who has spent time in a high-security New York prison. With AIDS and mild dementia, he nevertheless sought out a therapist to discuss two issues: the the negative reactions he encounters outside of prison and "getting ready" to continue life with AIDS. He could understand but had trouble coping with staff reaction at a rooming house he now lived in. "You see, I was always the mediator in prison. People had differences, they'd come to me. We'd talk. I'd try to fix them up. When people heard I was sick, they protected me. Only once somebody wanted to hurt me. But my friends told him, 'no, you don't try anything with Mikey.' " This gentle man, whose crimes were nonviolent, was a conciliator, but could find no reconciliation outside of prison. Now he had AIDS, and was doubly scorned. His task as he saw it was to "make up for a lot of things, and let people get to know me, and then they'll like me."

Another drug user is John, the black sheep of his South Bronx family. When seen in an outpatient clinic, he was using drugs although he had been detoxed during a previous AIDS-related hospitalization. Upon discharge, John found himself stressed. "I went back to my crutch. It's what I know, and I went back to it," he explained. Now, he too was seeking help for his drug use, but also for his parents who were elderly. His father suffered from Alzheimer's Disease and hardly knew other family members. His mother, who had high blood pressure, continued to care lovingly for her spouse. John was concerned for his parents and his therapy goal was to learn how he could lessen the burden on his mother. John was hospitalized again, for an AIDS-related illness. On the third day of that hospitalization he received a phone call from his mother: His father had died suddenly. He then wanted to deal with his bereavement.

Both Mikey and John benefited from psychotherapy. One did not halt his occasional drug use. But the psychotherapeutic relationship and some of the content made it easier to deal with life. Neither these men nor other drug users can be treated by practitioners who view them as stereotypical members of an unwashed and degenerate crowd. To allow oneself to know the individual is to allow oneself to be taught that there is much to be gained from working with this group.

THERAPY CONSIDERATIONS

Traditional psychotherapy rules might have eliminated John as a possible client because of his continuing drug use. Blanket prohibitions against treating persons who continue to use drugs will eliminate many of this population from access to therapy. To avoid dismissing such clients, a careful triage of the potential client and a careful consideration of the limitations of the therapist and the context in which one works must be conducted.

Assessment of Motivation

A good first question, in any setting, is "Why do you seek services?" As IVDUs often come to therapy because they are referred, it is useful to discriminate between the referring clinician's reasons for therapeutic work and those of the prospective client. Batki, Sorensen, Faltz, and Madover (1988) observed:

> A common situation is one in which the health professional has been quite anxious to bring the AIDS patient into treatment because of substance abuse or public health concerns. However, often the clinician who is making a referral may be more concerned about substance abuse than is the patient, who may attempt to deny this problem. (p. 5)

It is important to inquire in detail regarding the prospective client's reasons for appearing.

Therapists seem to have an inordinate fear of being "conned," and look with skeptical eye upon those with criminal records or drug histories. Yet, unless there is coercion by the criminal justice system to enter a psychotherapy program, little is to to be gained from conning one's way into a psychotherapy program. Perhaps the therapist can "absorb" some conning, observing it and learning while also determining if psychotherapeutic benefit is possible. At the most basic level, one has to have a realistic assessment of the potential client's motivation to seek out a therapᵤ utic contact. These clients have the best of motives to end drug use: Staying alive.

More skepticism is required if the client believes, by joining a psychotherapy program, he or she will receive prescriptions for drugs to quell anxiety ("nerves") or other negative moods. Sometimes the potential client knows exactly what pharmaceuticals are needed. A fairly large debate over the psychiatric treatment of these individuals already exists, and can hardly be settled here. Some psychiatrists have taken a behavioral tack, making prescriptions of anxiolytics or other medications contingent upon behavior or, looking at it another way, using the prescriptions as operants to shape behaviors. The client receives the benzodiazepines or other medication only with behavior change, or continuing participation in psychotherapy, as reported by another mental health professional.

Other reasons for entering psychotherapy at this time include: belief that death is imminent and certain matters need to be "cleaned up;" belief that psychotherapy is part of medical treatment and can contribute to increased well-being, or that participation in psychotherapy may excuse continuing drug use.

Assessment of Preexisting Psychopathology

The assessment of a potential client with a history of drug use must acknowledge the high rates of mood and personality disorders in this population. A survey of 501 persons seeking assistance with substance abuse problems found that 78% had a lifetime psychiatric disorder, other than substance abuse, while 65% had a current mental disorder when they sought help (Ross, Glaser, & Germanson, 1988). These researchers said the most common lifetime disorders (excluding generalized anxiety disorder) were sociopathic personality disorder (41.0% of the sample), phobias (25.7%), psychosexual dysfunctions (24.1%), major depression (20.3%), and dysthymia (9.2%). The average number of lifetime diagnoses was 4.8 per subject; the average number of current diagnoses was 3.5 per subject. Ross, Glaser, and Germanson (1988) also noted that those who abused both alcohol and other drugs were the most psychiatrically impaired.

Other researchers diagnosed personality disorders in about 50% of a sample of 74 cocaine and 43 opioid dependent men (Malow, West, Williams, & Sutker, 1989). These percentages are likely low due to the exclusion of polysubstance abusers. Thirty-five percent of the opiate users and 6% of cocaine users were judged to have borderline personality disorder. Twenty-one percent of opioid users were found to have antisocial personality disorder, compared to 12% in the cocaine group.

Therapy Goals and Themes

What are realistic psychotherapy goals? In drug treatment programs, abstinence from controlled substances is the paramount goal. With HIV-infected persons having a history of drug use, other goals, both long- and shortterm, may be more realistic and valuable. The primary goal, of course, is improvement of quality of life, which is possible. Within this general goal are specific matters such as education regarding the medical aspects of HIV with the goal of increasing compliance; gaining access to community resources; practicing safer sex and needle cleaning, thus protecting others; improving the relationships with spouse, children, and other family members; dealing with bereavement; and the therapeutic goals of reconciliation and coming to terms.

It is not unusual for an IVDU to understand that the illness means his or her life is foreshortened. In order not to die a "junkie," this IVDU may turn to an available counselor to "clean up" problems that may include relationships with friends and family, continuing drug use, antisocial behaviors such as theft, and concerns about dying.

Many, however, who express these concerns when severely stressed (such as during a hospitalization for HIV disease), will fail to appear for therapy when the stress is alleviated. Other who start therapy may soon disappear.

This is in conformance with what I call the "unholy trinity" of drug-user dynamics: Impulse-control problems, urge to escape, and denial.

Impulse-control problems are illustrated by the statement, "I want it when I want it." One client expressed this in justifying unprotected sex with a woman friend: "I wanted to have sex and I didn't have a condom." He was oblivious to the notion that one could have been soon obtained; he could not delay gratification. Another example is that of the hospitalized methadone user whose dose is delayed. This person may harass staff or manipulatively threaten such serious behaviors as suicide. This low tolerance for frustration can severely task health care providers' tolerances for frustration.

The urge to escape is often articulated as a need for independence, especially from societal and caregivers' expectations and requirements. One hospitalized patient said, "I know I'm sick but I don't want to stay in the hospital because they are always telling me what to do." Clinically, this may resemble and be founded in schizoid-like intolerance of close relationships, sociopathic intolerance of structures of any sort, or borderline instability.

The third aspect of the unholy trinity, denial, may severely compromise the client's health care. Batki, Sorensen, Faltz, and Madover (1988) warned of a "dual, interactive system of denial" which allows the person to continue drug use

> in an attempt to cope with his physical discomfort or psychological distress of his illness. Furthermore, the presence of medical problems may provide a 'reason' for the addict to use drugs. Finally, continuing drug use and the lifestyle associated with it can be seen as a way in which patients seek to maintain the illusion of health. (p. 7)

Is Abstinence Required?

Traditional guidelines would require us to ensure that clients are drug-free before entering into a therapeutic relationship. Strict drug-counseling guidelines usually require periodic random urine screens to detect illicit substances. These guidelines have value if the primary goal of psychotherapy is to maintain drug-free living. However, with AIDS-related psychotherapy, we may want to consider the cost to the client of a psychotherapy contract that he or she cannot adhere to, versus benefits that may be realized over the longterm from a less ambitious contract. While working on shortterm goals, we may also work toward the longterm goal of encouraging substance abuse treatment. It may be that the therapeutic relationship can help produce motivation for treatment.

Faltz and Madover (1987), suggested,

> Someone who is in strong denial about a substance abuse problem may simultaneously be having great difficulty accepting the diagnosis of AIDS. For this reason it is better not to bring up the subject of substance abuse treatment until the patient has had a couple of weeks or so to begin to absorb the impact of the AIDS diagnosis. (p. 64)

Psychotherapist's Ability to Contract

Two aspects may interfere with the therapist's participation. First, unsupervised or unanalyzed negative feelings about drug use should disqualify one from the relationship. Second, the practitioner has to assess his or her competence as well as the capability of the practitioner's institution or setting in treating persons with drug problems.

Working in a general hospital without a drug program, a psychotherapist was approached by a man who said he was on methadone, but nevertheless "shot up" because he liked the street life. Once convicted and imprisoned for armed robbery, the potential client said he had access to a gun and $6,000 cash in a family safe. The family did not know he had the combination. Because there was imminent danger of use of a weapon, the therapist required the potential client to disclose the situation to his father, which occurred in the second session. But, because the drug use continued out of control and the hospital provided no specialized drug-related services, a referral was made to other institutions. It was the therapist's judgment that the potential client needed a "holding environment" which would provide specialized dawn-to-dusk day care, including counseling and psychiatric services, to contain the client's runaway habit.

If the therapist opts to work with a drug user, safeguards must be in place. Waivers of confidentiality must be required so the therapist can exchange information with the client's methadone program, physician, and other caregivers. Other questions must be considered: Is the person receiving adequate HIV-related care, and is a referral to a specialty center possible? Are community drug-treatment programs available? Would the client benefit from participation in a self-help program, such as Alcoholics Anonymous or Narcotics Anonymous? In many Narcotics Anonymous chapters, however, persons on methadone are not allowed to "share." This rule is changing, however, and may erode more quickly if HIV-positive clients are urged to confront the chapter or form their own chapters.

Availability of Supportive Caregivers

While a former drug user may be noncompliant or difficult to motivate, many have more highly functioning family members who are concerned about the client's well-being and willing to be enlisted in the patient's care. Their inclusion in the treatment plan provides additional significant leverage. Of course, this cannot be accomplished if the client insists that family members not know about his or her HIV-status. The reluctance to tell others, as already noted, may have more to do with the client's self-protection against shame or additional rejection than with protection of others.

Availability of Community Drug Treatment

One reason mental health practitioners shun substance abusers is shortage of adequate treatment programs in the community (American Health Consultants, 1989). Even if a therapist convinces a client to participate in a treatment program, there may be a long waiting list.

In one case, a practitioner began calling detoxification facilities on behalf of a client and became frustrated when someone willing to answer questions could not be found. How much more frustrated the client must be! Anticipatory management is key here. Many communities have, at some level, a clearinghouse for drug-treatment information. Practitioners should have some knowledge of their community's public and private substance abuse treatment centers.

One complication of methadone treatment is that many drug-counseling programs provide little, inadequate, or no counseling, and some centers have been opened just to provide the medication. Some settings that do provide counseling hire persons with little or no counseling training, then provide little education and supervision, and in general have poor quality control. Methadone programs vary in philosophy. Some tend to maintain clients on small doses of methadone indefinitely, while others seek drug-free status as quickly as possible. It helps to investigate the program before referral.

Working with the IVDU client requires reassessment of one's goals as a therapist. If one cannot afford one or two Medicaid clients who may be noncompliant, then the client–therapist match maybe a poor one. But if it is affordable and if one wants to be useful to those who have been psychologically embattled most of their lives, learn how to treat very difficult cases, gain knowledge about the disaffected, and be professionally challenged, then a client with a history of IVDU may be rewarding.

PREPARATIONS

Before taking on such a client, the private practitioner should take several preparatory steps including reviewing the literature, familiarizing himself or herself with the public issues, and learning responses to noncompliance.

Literature Review

Research and other theoretical writings are now providing more insight into the behaviors of intravenous drug users. Unfortunately or fortunately, there are many literatures on drug use. Somewhat overlapping but also distinct are the literatures of psychiatry, which tend to focus on biomedical aspects and drug therapies; psychology, which tend to use animal models and theoretical arguments for substance use (Fowles, 1988); and the substance abuse specialty literature, which tends to be "softer" in that it is more anecdotal, experience-based, and descriptive, with conclusions less likely to be based on scientifically designed research.

Another literature is the psychodynamic, represented by Khantzian, a psychiatrist who has suggested that heroin use is an attempt to cope with problems that include emotional pain, stress, and dysphoria (Khantzian, Mack, & Schatzberg, 1974). He has also suggested that drug users are self-medicators, with the choice of drug dependent on the psychopharmacological action of the drug and their dominant painful feelings (1985). Khantzian's thinking allows for a more compassionate view of substance abusers. However, others suggest that self-medicators are, at most, a subset of the drug-using population (Brown, Ridgely, Pepper, Levine, & Ryglewicz, 1989). See also Vaillant (1975) for a psychodynamic view of sociopathy in substance abusers.

Familiarity with Public Issues

Another useful preparation for working with drug-using clients is familiarization with the public debate—which can have unique aspects depending on the community—around these issues. Often these debates reveal much about community biases regarding drug users. The issues that may promote debates include methadone-use philosophy (lifetime maintenance versus gradual detoxification) and extent of methadone treatment, use of street programs to alert drug users to HIV, needle distribution programs, and decriminalization of drug use. It is also eye-opening to witness the community debate when a drug-treatment center is planned.

Responses to Noncompliance

Some IVDUs' noncompliance with institutional—such as hospital or treatment program—rules, lack of cooperation, and unreliability often cause intense negative feelings in service providers. In hospitals, inevitably someone demands that the noncompliant patient be discharged.

Institutional rules can be seen in several ways. Many regulations are created to protect both the client and staff. Some, however, may be seen as an institutional internalization of biases against certain clients. This may be found in the rules or procedures that seem, without good rationale, to militate against serving the considerable needs of the IVDU client. An example is a hospital's reluctance to consider the special pain needs of a drug using client (see Selwyn, 1989). When the patient leaves the hospital against medical advice to find pain relief on the street, hospital staff blame the patient, rather than consider their role in the episode.

The first consideration in serving a noncompliant client is whether the problem resides in the service providers. Often the issue is as simple as lack of specialized knowledge. For example, does the clinician react negatively to the methadone user being treated for tuberculosis who complains of withdrawal-like symptoms and requests more methadone? If so, the clinician may be unaware of a 1976 article by Kreek, Garfield, Gutjarh, and Guisti that indicated rifampin, commonly used to treat tuberculosis, may dramatically increase methadone excretion and result in withdrawal symptoms. Selwyn (1989) noted this and other possible drug interactions with methadone, including phenytoin (Tong, Pond, Kreek, Jaffery, & Benowitz, 1981), phenobarbital, diazepam, and desipramine (Kreek, 1983).

Another consideration is whether there is a reluctance to rethink certain procedures and rules, so clients can be treated as they are, rather than as service providers would like them to be. A hidden message behind a reluctance to change is "We want you to be like us, then we'll treat you." The task of clinicians is to understand clients' limitations and design treatment programs that address these limitations.

Anticipation, education, and supervision can ameliorate many if not most of the negative feelings regarding drug users. Realistic anticipation allows you to know what noncompliant behaviors may occur and allows you to stipulate limits. Education may point to new understandings of the plight of the drug user. Supervision, which is necessary to understand and work through negative feelings, will help a practitioner provide better service, as well as encourage personal growth.

15
Worried Well

John, a svelte, pleasant, gay man came to an HIV-testing clinic because he was sure he was HIV positive. In fact, he said, he had been treated with Mycelex for oral thrush, and he now was simply seeking confirmation for what he already strongly suspected.

Because he was so anxious, he was referred to the clinic's psychologist for additional assessment. After the assessment, John agreed to enter postscreening psychotherapy to help deal with the expected result.

In another case, a man claiming to be a minister went to the emergency room of a hospital run by his denomination. He explained that he was a missionary from South America, had contracted and been treated for AIDS there, but came to the United States for additional treatment. Because this man was well-spoken and authoritative about AIDS-related conditions, he was hospitalized and a regimen of zidovudine was begun. While the workup was being done, the minister approached patients with offers of spiritual counseling.

Neither John nor the minister were HIV-positive (and it turned out the minister was an imposter). John, who continued in psychotherapy, was believed to have hypochondriasis, or hypochondriacal neurosis, with AIDS a focus of his concerns. It is likely the "minister" could be diagnosed with Munchausen syndrome, now called factitious disorder with physical symptoms (APA, 1987).

In the early years of AIDS, John and the "minister" may have been described as "worried well," an undifferentiated category of individuals anxious about the illness and having difficulty containing their fears.

Symptoms prominent among the worried well may include anxiety that ranges from mild to extreme, ruminative thinking or intrusive obsessional thoughts, vague somatic concerns, delusions, inability to be reassured, and, possibly, histories of psychiatric disorders that have taken an AIDS focus.

More experience with these individuals has suggested that the informal category contains two subgroups: Persons with legitimate concerns and those who can be reassured by facts of transmission and testing, and others whose AIDS-related concerns and behaviors are not alleviated or abated by medical information and negative HIV tests. Those in the first group can be easily treated; those in the second group, who are not responsive to education and negative test results, will be the focus of this chapter.

Because those in the second subgroup of the worried well may have a more serious pathology, as do the two men described, careful psychological assessment and diagnosis should be routine for differentiation and treatment. Also included routinely should be communication with the client's physician, who can confirm the medical aspects of a client's situation.

ASSESSING CONCERNS

A first step is the assessment of the concern. Persons who may have a reasonable basis for anxiety include those who suspect that a former or current sex partner engaged in risk behaviors, know a former sex partner is now ill or dead, have been sexually active in an urban area with a large number of HIV-infected persons, or had a transfusion before mid-1985. Those more likely to have an unfounded reason for anxiety include those concerned about sexual encounters before 1980 and those anxious despite a longstanding monogamous relationship. Of course, the assessment picture is complicated by the possibility that those who express AIDS-related anxiety are untruthfully denying risk behaviors. Some present with vague physical complaints that, they say, were given short shrift by their physicians.

The initial interview should conclude with the client signing a waiver of confidentiality, enabling the therapist to obtain information from the physician. While the therapist does not require copies of medical records, a phone discussion should include inquiries about HIV testing and results, the client's psychiatric and drug-use history, and doctor's assessment of the physical complaints.

Does Reassurance Work?

A second step in assessment and treatment is the attempt to educate and, thereby, reassure. For example, a person in a longstanding monogamous relationship or someone worried about infection due to a few casual contacts is normally reassured by facts about HIV transmission and its history in the community.

Anonymous HIV testing is another means of reassurance. If anxiety and ruminations are disruptive and the chances of infection small, the client may choose to opt for testing. A negative result should alleviate the anxiety. (A positive result removes the client from the category of worried well.) The test itself is always a cause for anxiety, no matter how insignificant the potential risk. The anxiety, which spans the time from consideration it until test results are obtained, can be provoked by the testing process, which includes blood drawing in a formal medical setting.

If a person declines testing, the therapist must assess the legitimacy of the reasons. Legitimate concerns may include the unavailability of anonymous testing or lack of confidentiality in a small community. However, if the client reports disruptive agitation or rumination and either declines anonymous testing or is unwilling to make efforts to be tested, such as travelling to another community, then a more serious psychopathology may be indicated.

Other Differentiating Variables

This reluctance to resolve the issue through test results is one of several variables that separate the merely worried from those with psychopathology. Others include:

- Inability to be convinced.

The worried well person may have engaged in risk behaviors and will consider HIV testing, albeit anxiously. This client is reassured by a negative test result and returns to normal functioning. The more seriously psychiatrically involved person may have had one or several HIV tests with negative results, but remains unconvinced. Usually, a plausible reason is given for the doubt: "I had unsafe sex less than 6 months ago," one may hear. Or, "I'm probably one of those persons who takes a long time to get antibodies." In fact, even if tests are repeated, some *will not* be reassured by available facts—a hallmark of a more severe condition. Others with serious psychopathology may sabotage the possibility of having a conclusive test by continuing to engage in unsafe behaviors that effectively prevent closing the window of nondetectability.

- Vague or nonexistent history of risk behaviors.

The worried person may have engaged in risk behaviors or had a transfusion, but the delusional person could be unable to describe or date them. Descriptions of such behaviors may be vague, with unverifiable suspicions expressed regarding sex partners. These typically take the form of, "I just didn't trust him or her." An unwillingness to verify suspicions is also cause for concern. For example, if one asks if the suspected sex partner is ill and the client says no effort was made to find out, despite the current AIDS anxiety, then psychopathology may be indicated.

• History of concerns about other illnesses.

A person who may be hypochondriacal may have been previously concerned about other illnesses or symptoms prior to the onset of AIDS concern. Inquiries should be made about concerns about other illnesses predating AIDS.

• History of obsessive compulsive disorder symptoms, including washing or other rituals.

Symptoms noted in DSM-III-R (APA, 1987) include recurrent, persistent ideas and attempts to suppress or neutralize these thoughts, as well as intentional, repetitive behaviors designed to neutralize some discomfort.

• History of excessive anxiety, generally, along with the physiologic symptoms noted in DSM-III-R—the sort that may lead one to a generalized anxiety disorder diagnosis.
• Other symptoms of mental disorder, such as delusions.

DIAGNOSTIC CONSIDERATIONS

If reassurance and repeated HIV testing fail to allay symptoms, the following diagnostic possibilities should be considered:

• Obsessive compulsive disorder, especially with a history of previous concerns and rituals.

Almost one third of a sample of obsessive compulsive patients have incorporated AIDS into their rituals and beliefs, reported Rapoport (1990). She noted that AIDS may be used as a rationale for washing behaviors that preceded the AIDS concerns.

• Delusional (paranoid) disorder.

One diagnostic criterion is nonbizarre delusions, including having a disease. While not providing a specific diagnosis, Cochran and Mays (1989) described a 38-year-old woman with a number of somatic complaints that included fatigue, weight loss, swollen glands, fever, and sweats. Telephone calls to AIDS information groups provided information that helped convince her she had AIDS. With assessment, Cochran discovered the patient was suffering from a delusional process.

• Hypochondriasis (or hypochondriacal neurosis).

This includes diagnostic criteria of preoccupation with the fear of having or the belief that one has a serious disease, and with appropriate medical evaluation failing to find a medical disorder that can account for the symptoms described.

- Factitious disorder.

Several case accounts are available, including the one of the HIV-negative, bogus minister (see Bialer & Wallack, 1990). Diagnostic criteria include a psychological need to assume a sick role and intentional production or feigning of physical symptoms.

- Somatization disorder.

Typical complaints that raise fear of AIDS include diarrhea and other gastrointestinal symptoms; shortness of breath; and pseudoneurological symptoms such as amnesia, difficulty swallowing, muscle weakness, vision problems, and pseudoseizures. DSM-III-R lists seven symptoms as a screening device; the presence of two or more may point to this diagnosis.

These considerations will aid a clinician to make a sophisticated diagnosis of a client who presents as worried well and to formulate an appropriate treatment plan, ranging from education and support to psychiatric treatment for a major mental illness. AIDS concerns may be only the presenting symptom.

16
Spirituality

Last year, I was with a woman who was dying of cancer. She was relatively young, with lots of plans and hopes for the future. Her husband visited her daily, and she had a young adult daughter who was finding her mother's impending death particularly painful. One day, in great anguish, the young woman said to her father, "How can God let this happen?" And her father, a simple man with little book knowledge or theological training, replied: "Look, God doesn't like this any more than we do."

God doesn't like AIDS any more than we do. . . . And God is neither cause of our suffering nor some kind of divine rescuer who will swoop down and save us. (p. 2)

In this unpublished eulogy to a man who died of AIDS, Conforti (1987) describes a God who "is always with us in the process as co-suffering, compassionate presence. . . . God lives within us and among us. . . . He is there where we are there for one another" (p. 2).

Facing the mystery and suffering of HIV illness, both client and therapist may turn to religion, spirituality, and concepts of God in their efforts to find solace, understanding, and emotional healing. Often, the issues of connection to a greater reality; blame, shame, or guilt based on religious beliefs; and the role of God become prominent issues in psychotherapy. Although some will continue their earnest disbelief, one also sees in HIV-positive persons the full range of religious beliefs, practices, and motivations, including new inquiries and practices candidly described as a "hedging of bets" and sincere identifications with long-ago learned or newly intuited matters of faith. One may hear longings for connections to old traditions, and searches for new senses of meaning. These efforts can provide solace, a sense of belonging, and connection to a larger reality, or they can create new emotional hurts or remind clients of old strictures and messages of guilt and punishment.

One does not do justice to any belief by accepting it without question or study. Any dogma or collection of beliefs must be strong enough to withstand scrutiny and is honored by conscious and considered, rather than by thought-less, acceptance.

Understanding a Client's Religious Feelings

To understand a client's religious feelings, it may be helpful to inquire about the religious life of the patient in the context of pre-HIV life and culture. Is the religious practice new since the client learned of HIV status, or is it renewed? How does this practice fit into the context of the client's life? Is the person wearing a Catholic rosary as a sign of a new religion-based resolve but continuing to use drugs? Did the belief and dedication to a religion provide solace before HIV?

If the therapist is mystified or made uncomfortable by a client's religious discussions, it may also be useful to learn about the religious tradition that contributes to the client's perceptions. A consultation with a carefully chosen clergy person of that tradition would be useful. The person should be willing to describe a full range of attitudes and theological scholarship regarding the client's alternative lifestyles that are extant in the denomination's discourse. For example, within the Roman Catholic church in the United States, a wide variety of theological views exist regarding homosexuality, from outright con-demnation to acceptance. Also, Melton's (1989) collection of church docu-ments on AIDS may provide some insight into the denomination's public stance. If the therapist remains uncomfortable with religious themes, the client can be urged to consult a religious or spiritual adviser.

NEGATIVE MESSAGES BASED ON RELIGION

Unfortunately, the public discourse about AIDS includes religiously based statements that AIDS is a divine punishment (Steinfels, 1989). Some refer to a person with AIDS as a victim of the wrath of God, or WOG. This stance seems illogical on its face: What did children with AIDS do to deserve this "punishment?" Now, many denominations have issued public statements that urge conciliation and compassion, while not necessarily approving alternate lifestyles or sexual preferences (Melton, 1989). Unfortunately, many times the denomination's ambivalent feelings are described as "We love the sinner but hate the sin." This does little to mollify individuals who do not view their sexual activities as sinful.

But the condemnatory spirit behind statements such as WOG and "hate the sin" have been internalized by many HIV-positive persons and transformed into a self-condemnatory and intrapunitive attitude. Using reasoning based in religious tenets, a client may justify shame, guilt, and intrapunitive feelings and behaviors. Sometimes friends and family too may use threats of punishment by God to urge conversion to or realignment with family beliefs. This may be the product of a genuine faith, familial guilt and shame, or a fantasy that new religiosity may lead to cure.

Moreover, many believe a powerful God has foresaken them. "Why can't God rescue my son. He's done it with others. Why can't he do it with my child," cried one mother of a PWA. This woman believed God can intervene and chose not to. Somewhere herein is the uncomforting image of God as a punishing, vengeful Lord, à la Cotton Mather. It raises the spectre of a people at the deity's mercy: God as the source or controller of AIDS. If the plague is sent and not removed, is this not a sign of guilt or disfavor?

In psychological terms, this type of thinking is known as blaming the victim. When a random event, such as an assault or illness, occurs, people tend to say, "Oh, it occurred because the victim didn't play it safe." The victim dared to walk at night or was a homosexual. This alleviates anxiety stirred by these events, because the attribution is that the victim caused the trouble. If one avoids the unsafe act—if one is virtuous—then one will remain safe. Another possibility is that it is easier to blame the victim because one fears being angry with God. This can result in intrapunitive behavior, depression, and angry outbursts.

In the AIDS discussion, subtle blaming of the victim is often revealed by use of the phrase "innocent victims of AIDS." This usually refers to children and those infected by blood transfusions. The noninnocents, or "guilty" victims are gay men or needle users. This application of guilt and innocence may be abetted by religiously based concepts of innocence and blame.

RELIGIOSITY VERSUS RELIGIOUS EXPERIENCE

Many of the condemnatory and punitive messages are based on interpretations unleavened by mercy and compassion. These tend especially to mark beliefs and activities based in religiosity rather than spirituality. It is useful to differentiate between religiosity and religious experience—including use of symbol and ritual—that spring from our human experience. It is also helpful to distinguish between religiosity and spirituality.

By religiosity is meant a stereotypically patterned, unquestioning following of rules or "walking through the paces" concerned primarily with external practice. "Acting religious" may be part of a client's or caregiver's bargaining process: "For two rosaries, God will give me. . . . ." Little or no thought is given to understanding the derivations of external practice because, after all, only the externals are important. Moreover, fear of further retribution requires the individual to avoid questioning, exploring, or disagreeing with beliefs or practice. To the therapist, this type of person may appear much like someone with an obsessive personality disorder: overly conscientious, scrupulous, and inflexible. The beliefs and practices seem to have a life of their own, quite apart from relationship with a Creator or spiritual beliefs.

Religiosity, even New Age religiosity, seems also to lack a realistic view of life. One HIV-positive psychotherapy client, who also had a lover dying of AIDS, talked about those who led a New Age-type religious meeting he and his lover attended.

> I asked him if I and Paul had AIDS. And he consulted his Lama—he was channeling—and he said, "No, AIDS had not touched anyone in the room." And there we sat, Paul and I, and we knew we had the virus. This guy had to always be positive, but that was bullshit.

Contrast religiosity with a person's finding religious meaning in a system of symbols that spring naturally from and are authentic to one's life. These symbols may include God as a nurturing father or mother who provides solace; heaven as symbolic of a place of peace (as opposed to a physical space where there are cottages, lakes, and ice cream parlors); or the sense of unity with one another, and God as a unifying concept. In this concept, ritual, too, is an authentic outward expression of humanness. Rather than practices superimposed on individuals, ritual in this sphere springs from common experience and, if you will, collective unconscious. To name several examples, consider handshakes, embraces, the Hasidics' dance with the torah on the holiday of Simhath Torah, and the use of water in ritual. In these are contained religious experiences.

Spirituality, on the other hand, may not even be deity-centered. It may be an inner-generated, thoughtful, and sometimes skeptical search—a process rather than a product—for universal connections, with no *quid pro quo* from a higher power sought or intended. If the spirituality is God-centered, that God is a benevolent, generous, and caring deity who holds others blameless and is not to blame. Some believe that there is deity in all of us, and is not specific to one person, place, or time.

To those with this type of spiritual bent, the manifestation of God's love is found in relationships devoid of blame, acrimony, condescension, or withholding—whether at Catholic Mass, at Sabbath services, with a therapist, in a family gathering, or with friends in a hospital room. Where charity and love are, God is also, as a hymn suggests. Any other presentation seems devoid of charity, a counterfeit.

HEALING ROLES OF RELIGION

Within these understandings, religion and spirituality can have many roles, none being punitive or contributory to self-hate. In the face of illness, religion can be an element in attaining connection and reconnection. It can promote homecoming—a reconnection to roots, felt profoundly and yet inexpressible.

It can provide psychic space, within which a person can find opportunities to question and build one's own belief system. Moreover, spirituality can foster forgiveness and healing.

Forgiveness is not meant in a moralistic sense, for being immoral or "bad." Rather, religion can help the ill person forgive God for not rescuing or playing *deus ex machina* (Clark, 1986) and forgive the universe for the craziness and tragedy of the situation. In forgiving life and forgiving God, a sense of blame is laid to rest and one forgives himself or herself as well.

By healing is meant what some may regard as "salvation." Not a physical cure, salvation is often described as profound self-acceptance, in which an individual experiences himself or herself as viewed and loved by God simply as he or she is. With this acceptance by God, a client accepts all.

PART 5

RESOURCES

17
Creative Rethinking
of Service Delivery

On a snowy December day, a Manhattan physician who works with hospital-ized PWAs was discussing a phone call he had received. A man with severe AIDS dementia came to the psychiatric emergency room of a Brooklyn hospi-tal. Someone there decided the patient did not have a psychiatric disorder and should go to the medical emergency room. In the medical emergency room, someone decided the patient was really a psychiatric case. A hospital social worker called the physician, desperate to find a safe place for the PWA.

The AIDS situation in New York City, and in every community with a significant number of PWAs, portends a crisis for the 1990s. The worst-case scenario now is one of warehousing—hospitalization of PWAs in large wards, with only occasional physicians' visits and care provided by relatively un-skilled technicians and orderlies. Warehousing seems extremely plausible in light of increasing numbers of PWAs; declining absolute numbers of doctors and nurses; relatively fewer health care providers who want to work with PWAs due to preconceptions, risks, and little financial incentive; and no societal will to make the changes and investments necessary to respond to the AIDS crisis.

It is clear to most observers that until the medical miracle of a cure arrives, the medical aspects of the AIDS epidemic alone will outpace all traditional attempts at health care service delivery. They already have, in cities such as New York, where governmental agencies failed to organize and integrate services. It is also clear that the old systems, built on the medical model, cannot begin to treat the psychosocial and psychopolitical aspects of AIDS: commu-nity instability (Wallace, 1988), poverty, drug abuse, and stigma among those on a long list.

191

Creative "whole systems" (medical, political, and psychosocial) planning must occur elsewhere—Tallahassee, Des Moines, or Dayton, for example—with acknowledgement of the errors and failures of other communities. A dedication must be made to creative planning in health care delivery that may involve whole new ways of seeing problems and solutions—paradigm shifts, such as those described by Kuhn (1970). Required now are persons who can think in new ways and who have the patience and stamina to understand that the fight against this epidemic will be a marathon, rather than a sprint.

Few professionals are better able to make more knowledgeable and creative contributions than mental health service providers, who are blessed with compassion, intelligence, and a holistic view of the patient that integrates the medical, psychological, and spiritual. The following suggestions may be useful if one feels that providing psychotherapy is not enough, and that work needs to be done to change systems: to provide additional services, seek additional knowledge, restructure service delivery systems, and prepare for the 1990s.

Systems versus Closeup Views

The first challenge in creative thinking with AIDS is the same dilemma experienced by the photographer who has a wide-angle lens to capture the broad view, as well as a macro lens to focus close up on a small and narrow area. Which lens does one choose? In AIDS work, few practitioners have both lenses. Researchers, with the wide-angle lenses of group studies, can well capture the "bigger picture." Their products are often found in technical journals or in the proceedings of conferences sponsored by think tanks or governmental agencies (see LeVee, 1989, for example). But few researchers have the "hands-on" experience that captures the distinctions and complexities of individual cases. Clinicians are focused on individuals, and often are too specialized to participate in the broad view.

With AIDS-related planning, one must both understand the larger, systemic picture, and plan small, finely focused changes in delivery systems. The larger focus is provided by reading and by talking with researchers. The narrow focus is provided by clinical experience. The clinician, especially one who works closely with local systems, quickly learns what resources are lacking and why problems appear and can often conceptualize solutions.

Making Ideas into Reality

The following considerations are offered to help practitioners turn ideas into practical proposals.

1. Create the Idea for Change

This is not complicated or magical, but is often just a spontaneously conceived and simple idea for significant change. It is often spoken in the phrase, said so often, "Wouldn't it be better if. . . ." One example of a simple idea with potentially large implications was a hospital practitioner's observation, "Wouldn't it be better if family caregivers knew more about home care? That way, clients may get better care when they leave the hospital." That idea led to a grant proposal to fund home care training for PWAs' caregivers.

2. Search the Literature

You will want to learn three things. First, has your idea, or some permutation, been reported in AIDS work; second, has it been attempted in another medical area, such as cancer, kidney disease, or diabetes; third, what has your profession and other, related professionals, contributed.

A librarian who knows literature searches will simplify your task. Large university and medical school libraries now have specific AIDS-related databases. The *Compact Library: AIDS,* by the Medical Publishing Group is a collection of compact disks with a MEDLINE subset on AIDS as well as other information. It is updated quarterly. The Psychological Abstracts Information Services (PsycInfo) provides an AIDS-related bibliography as well as broader information. To find references, you must use words and phrases utilized by the service and contained in the database thesaurus.

In your search of what other professionals have contributed, you may find yourself using the *Cumulative Index to Nursing and Allied Health, Social Work Research and Abstracts,* or PsycInfo. Also, you may call a local education and training center (see Appendix) and the National AIDS Information Clearinghouse, which has librarians to help you find important documents.

When reading research reports, keep in mind that the actual work tends to be years old by the time of publication. Much of the "cutting edge" work is discussed in professional meetings long before publication. If possible, augment your reading with attendance at such conferences.

3. Operationalize

It was insufficient to say that home care training should be provided. "Operationalizing"—narrowly defining with sufficient detail the practical way changes should be made—"fleshed out" this training, or defined all its aspects, resulting in: a richly detailed training curriculum based on already existing home care training and the actual experiences of caregivers, a training schedule, and a research protocol to determine if the training was effective and helpful. Spare no details; they can always be deleted.

4. Formulate in a Few Pages and Circulate to Colleagues

This tests the waters, to determine whether the idea is practically and politically viable. It also begins building a coalition that will politically support the project. Ask for advice, comments, and names of others, including persons elsewhere, who may contribute. Determine if there is a researcher or a supervisor who will advise and support the project.

5. Investigate Funding Sources

Grants-seeking is quickly becoming a specialty. Persons who work in university settings may find that an administration office may have a grants specialist who can be consulted. Others may want to consult researchers who are already funded, foundations listings in libraries, and local foundations and funding agencies.

Federal agencies usually will fund only specific aspects of projects, and require quite sophisticated grant applications. Their processes are usually complex and time-consuming.

More likely sources of funds are either local foundations or those either AIDS-specific, such as the American Foundation for AIDS Research, or AIDS-interested. Foundations' AIDS interest changes, and you will need current information. The Robert Wood Johnson Foundation had generously funded grants for AIDS-related projects, but changed its focus in 1989.

6. Ask for Help With Expertise or Resources

The clinician who produced the home care training idea knew he did not have the grant-seeking expertise, but found a respected medical economics researcher, familiar with grants, who agreed to collaborate as did others in her department. This represented an ideal blend of wide-angle and narrow-focus practitioners. Contact local researchers and ask for advice and, if necessary, collaboration.

7. Do Not Become Discouraged

The best AIDS ideas are, by their nature, 3 to 5 years ahead of their time. Someone with a brilliant idea is likely way ahead of his or her time, and the rest will catch up, eventually. Unfortunately, however, eventually may be too late for too many.

The practitioner's efforts to deal with AIDS, whether in psychotherapy, research, or creative efforts to improve service delivery, are the noblest of efforts. In the face of an illness which is more daunting and more complicated than any we could imagine, many persons are providing their best efforts. These efforts, based in *caritas* and competence, are healing. Whether one does psychotherapy exclusively, combines therapy with research, or provides other services to HIV-positive persons, one participates in the noblest way in life.

Appendix
Resources

The following are offered as sources of information to augment your information and keep your knowledge current. The list is by no means all-encompassing. It includes prominent organizations, publishers, and federally funded training centers, among others. Some provide information free, others ask a donation or sell publications.

COMPUTER APPLICATIONS
FOR THE DISABLED

Apple Computer Inc.
Office of Special Education and Rehabilitation
Phone: (408) 974-7910
Access also available through authorized dealers. Extensive data base of computer applications and related organizations and publications for disabled persons.

AT&T National Special Needs Center
Phone: (800) 233-1222
Information on telephone equipment for disabled persons.

Closing the Gap
P.O. Box 68
Henderson, MN 56044
Phone: (612) 248-3294
Publisher of semimonthly tabloid with information on computer applications for persons with special needs. One issue yearly is a resource directory of hardware and software.

IBM National Support Center for Persons with Disabilities
Box 2150
Atlanta, GA 30005
Phone: (800) 426-2133
Provides information on utilization of computers for disabled persons.

JOURNAL PUBLISHERS

Current Science
1201 Locust St.
Philadelphia, PA 19107-9824
Phone: (800) 552-5866
Publishes the journal *AIDS*.

Medical Publishing Group
1440 Main St.
Waltham, MA 02154-1649
Phone: (617) 893-3800
A division of the Massachusetts Medical Society, this company publishes *AIDS Clinical Care,* reprints *Morbidity and Mortality Weekly Report,* publishes several AIDS-related books, and has two compact disk and computer communications products, the *Compact Library: AIDS* and *AIDS Knowledge Base,* Among its books is *The AIDS Knowledge Base* (Cohen, Sande, & Volberding, 1990) which I believe is the best compendium of technical medical information about HIV.

Raven Press
1185 Avenue of the Americas
New York, NY 10036
Publishes the *Journal of Acquired Immune Deficiency Syndromes.*

NEWSLETTER PUBLISHERS

American Health Consultants Inc.
60 Peachtree Park Dr. NE
Atlanta, GA 30309-1397
Phone: (404) 351-4523
Publishes *AIDS Alert,* and *AIDS Medical Report.*

CDC AIDS Weekly Subscription Office
P.O. Box 830409

Birmingham, AL 35283-0409
Phone: (800) 633-4931
(205) 991-6920
Publishes the weekly newsletter *CDC AIDS Weekly.*

Williams & Wilkins
PO Box 23291
Baltimore, MD 21203-9990
Publishes *ATIN: AIDS Targeted Information Newsletter,* which contains literature reviews.

ORGANIZATIONS

American Foundation for AIDS Research
1515 Broadway, Suite 3601
New York, NY 10036-8901
Phone: (212) 719-0033
Funds research projects and publishes several compendiums of information, including AIDS information resource and experimental treatment directories. Also sponsors *ATIN: AIDS Targeted Information Newsletter,* a compendium of abstracts and citations, and *AIDS Clinical Care,* a newsletter.

American Social Health Association
P.O. Box 13287
Research Triangle Park, NC 27709
ASHA publishes pamphlets and other information regarding sexually transmitted diseases, including AIDS, herpes, and genital warts.

Association of Asian/Pacific Community Health Organizations
310 Eighth St., Suite 310
Oakland, CA 94607
Phone: (405) 272-9536
Offers the first health education video on AIDS produced for and by Asians and Pacific Islanders, available in Cantonese, Korean, Samoan, Tagalog and Vietnamese. An English program guide is available.

Body Positive
P.O. Box 493
London W14 OTH UK
Telephone: 01-373 9124
A voluntary organization run by HIV-positive persons, with a telephone helpline open evenings.

Canadian AIDS Society
Suite 200
267 Dalhousie St.
Ottawa, Canada K1N 7E3
Phone: (613) 230-3580
A coalition of of community based groups fighting AIDS. Lists member organizations throughout Canada and has publications.

Gay Mens Health Crisis (GMHC)
129 W. 20th St.
New York, NY 10011-0022
Phone: (212) 807-6655
One of the first groups to coalesce around the epidemic. Wide range of quality publications available, as well as a hotline and social services. The booklet, *Medical Answers About AIDS,* alone is worth the price of a phone call.

Names Project
2362 Market St.
San Francisco, CA 94114
Phone: (800) USA-NAME
The Names Project is responsible for the intuitively appealing and touching quilt that memorializes those who died of AIDS.

National Council on Death and Dying
250 W. 57th St.
New York, NY 10107
Phone: (212) 246-6962
Two organizations recently merged to form one that has educational materials, a newsletter, Living Will forms, and a Living Will registry.

National Hemophilia Foundation
110 Greene St. Room 406
New York, NY 10012
Telephone: (212) 219-8180
FAX: (212) 966-9247
Provides informational publications regarding hemophilia and HIV. Will direct you to local chapters and regional comprehensive care centers for the person with hemophilia. Operates the hemophilia and AIDS/HIV Network for the Dissemination of Information, which offers publications, bibliographies, article reprints and other resources.

Project Inform
347 Dolores St.

Suite 301
San Francisco, CA 94110
Phones: National: (800) 822-7422; California: (800) 334-7422, San Francisco:
(415) 558-9051
Advocacy organization in San Francisco provides excellent bulletins and news
letters. They ask a donation upon receipt of the first mailing.

San Francisco AIDS Foundation
333 Valencia Street
San Francisco, CA 94101-6182
Phone: (415) 861-3397
Its *AIDS Educator* catalog includes more than 65 education and training tools,
with emphasis on cultural sensitivity and nonhomophobic language.

Terrence Higgins Trust Ltd.
52-54 Grays Inn Rd.
London WC1N 8JU
Phone: 01-242 1010
A charity that provides information and advice. Has a series of booklets and
a helpline.

UCSF AIDS Health Project
Box 0884
San Francisco, CA 94143-0884
Phone: (415) 476-6430
Publishes *Focus,* a highly informative newsletter, as well as books, video/audio
cassettes, and brochures.

POLITICAL ACTION GROUPS

ACT UP
496-A Hudson St.
Suite G4
New York, NY 10014
Phone: (212) 989-1114
This quasi-anarchistic organization provides well-researched information and
specializes in confrontative actions.

People with AIDS Coalition
31 W. 26th St.
Fifth floor
New York, NY 10010
Phone: (212) 532-0290

An organization of HIV-positive persons and others, providing information and sustenance.

PROFESSIONAL ORGANIZATIONS

American Psychiatric Association
AIDS Steering Committee
1400 K St. NW
Washington, DC 20005
Phone: (202) 682-6143
APA has published *A Psychiatrist's Guide to AIDS and HIV Disease,* a training program, computerized self-help test on the psychiatric aspects of AIDS, and training videos.

American Psychological Association
1200 17th St. N.W.
Washington, DC 20036
The association has an office on AIDS, which has a computerized AIDS Resource Network listing those who work with HIV disease, and a publication entitled *Psychology & AIDS Exchange.* Also, it publishes PsycINFO, a psychological abstracts information service, and the book *AIDS: Abstracts of the Psychological and Behavioral Literature* with updates.

Association of Nurses In AIDS Care
704 Stony Hill Rd.
Suite 106
Yardley, PA 19067
Phone: (215) 321-2371
Has annual meetings, local chapters, and publishes a journal.

New York State Psychological Association Task Force on AIDS
Barbara Eisold, PhD
285 Central Park West
New York, NY 10024
(See also American Psychological Association.)

Physicians Association for AIDS Care
101 W. Grand Ave.
Suite 200
Chicago, IL 60611
Phone: (312) 222-1326
Organization of physicians, provides AIDS-related programming via satellite to members.

REGIONAL EDUCATION
AND TRAINING CENTERS

The Health Resources and Services Administration of the U.S. Public Health Service has distributed millions of dollars in federal funds to train primary health care providers in diagnosis, treatment, and care of persons with HIV infection. As of October 1989, the following Education and Training Centers (ETCs) were providing a variety of services, including telephone information and seminars:

Site	*Service Area*
New York-Caribe AIDS/SIDA ETC 429 Shimkin Hall, Washington Square New York University New York, NY 10003 (212) 998-5335	New York City, Long Island, New Jersey, Puerto Rico, Virgin Islands
UW AIDS ETC 1001 Broadway Seattle, WA 98104 (206) 543-9750	Washington, Alaska, Montana, Idaho, Oregon
East Central AIDS ETC Area 300, 1314 Kinnear Road Columbus, OH 43212 (614) 292-1400	Ohio, Michigan, Kentucky, Tennessee
Western Aids ETC University of California—Davis California Area Health Education System 5110 East Clinton Way, Suite 115 Fresno, CA 93727-2098 (209) 252-2851	California (excluding 5 southern counties), Nevada, Arizona, Hawaii
Emory AIDS Training Network 735 Gatewood Road Atlanta, GA 30322 (404) 727-2929	Alabama, Florida, Georgia, North Carolina, South Carolina
Delta Region AIDS ETC LSU Sch. of Medicine, 1542 Tulane Ave. New Orleans, LA 70112 (504) 568-3855	Arkansas, Louisiana, Mississippi
Mountain Plains Regional AIDS ETC UCHSC Box A096, 4200 East 9th Ave. Denver, CO 80262 (303) 270-5885	North and South Dakota, Utah, Colorado, New Mexico, Nebraska, Kansas, Wyoming

Site	*Service Area*
Midwest AIDS ETC (MATEC) University of Illinois at Chicago 808 S. Wood Street (M/C 779) Chicago, IL 60612 (312) 996-1426	Iowa, Minnesota, Wisconsin, Illinois, Indiana, Missouri
Mid-Atlantic AIDS ETC University of Maryland at Baltimore 520 W. Lombard Street Baltimore, MD 21201 (301) 328-8334	Maryland, District of Columbia, Virginia, West Virginia, Delaware
New England AIDS ETC 55 Lake Avenue North Worchester, MA 01655 (508) 856-3255	Maine, Massachusetts, New Hampshire, Rhode Island, Vermont, Connecticut
USC ETC 1975 Zonal Avenue, KAM 200 Los Angeles, CA 90033 (213) 224-7038	Southern California counties of Los Angeles, Orange, Ventura, Riverside, San Bernardino
AIDS Regional ETCs for TX and OK Univ. of Texas Sch. of Public Health P. O. Box 20188 (RAS E-335) Houston, TX 77225 (713) 794-4075	Texas, Oklahoma
University of Pittsburgh AIDS ETC Graduate School of Public Health 130 De Soto Street Pittsburg, PA 15260 (412) 624-1895	Pennsylvania, upstate New York
Mid-Hudson Valley ETC Columbia Univ., Sch. of Public Health 600 West 168 Street, 7th Floor New York, NY 10032 (212) 305-3616	Hudson Valley area of upstate New York
Pennsylvania/New York ETC AIDS Training Center A-158 Albany Medical Center 47 New Scotland Avenue Albany, NY 12208 (518) 445-4675	Albany, NY area

SPECIAL INTEREST GROUPS

Women and AIDS Resource Network
P.O. Box 020525
Brooklyn, NY 11202
Phone: (718) 596-6007

Minority Task Force on AIDS
92 St. Nicholas Ave.
New York, NY 10026
Phone: (212) 749-2816

Association for Drug Abuse Prevention and Treatment
Phone: (212) 807-5560

Mothers of AIDS Patients
P.O. Box 89409
San Diego, CA 92138
Phone: (213) 450-6484 or 530-2109

SUBSTANCE ABUSE PUBLICATIONS

Manisses Communications Group, Inc.
Three Governor St.
P.O. Box 3357
Providence, RI 02906-0357
Publishes *The Brown University Digest of Addiction Theory and Application,*
a digest of addiction research found in more than 75 journals.

Substance Abuse Services
Wards 92 and 93
Department of Psychiatry
San Francisco General Hospital
1001 Potrero Ave.
San Francisco, CA 94110
Has a catalog of some 75 publications dealing with substance abuse available
for the price of photocopying. Also included are books and unpublished manu-
scripts.

TECHNICAL INFORMATION

National AIDS Information Clearinghouse.
U.S. Department of Health and Human Services
Public Health Service, Centers for Disease Control.

PO Box 6003
Rockville, MD 20850
Phone: (800) 458-5231
Fax: (301) 738-6616
TTY/TTD: (800) 243-7012
International Line: (301) 217-0023
Identifies organizations doing AIDS-related works; locates educational materials, offers citations and descriptions of resources for education of children, describes U.S. funding opportunities, and publishes information publications such as a conference calendar. Some information it provides is dated.

National Library of Medicine
Bethesda, MD 20894
Phone: (301) 496-6308
With a legislative mandate to create an AIDS-related data base, the library provides several online computer files, dealing with AIDS literature, information on clinical trials of drugs and vaccines, and resource organizations. It also produces a monthly bibliography and publishes a listing of health hotlines.

Agency for Health Care Policy and Research
Publications and Information Branch
18-12 Parklawn Bldg.
Rockville, MD 20857
Phone: (301) 443-4100
This branch of the U.S. Public Health Service funds research on problems related to quality, delivery, and costs of health services. It publishes *Research Activities*, a monthly newsletter, and notices of special research interests.

TELEPHONE INFORMATION LINES

American Social Health Association National Sexually Transmitted Diseases Hotline: (800) 227-8922.

Government of Quebec Toll Free Information Number: (800) 463-5656.

U.S. Public Health Service, Centers for Disease Control
U.S. statistics, age, race, and ethnic distribution, taped message: (404) 330-3020.

U.S. statistics, risk-group categories, taped message: (404) 330-3021.

U.S. state and metropolitan area statistics; estimates and projections, taped message: (404) 330-3022.

Cocaine Hotline: (800) COCAINE

National AIDS Hotline, service of the U.S. Public Health Service Centers for Disease Control: (800) 342-AIDS; in Spanish: (800) 344-SIDA.

Pediatric AIDS Hot Line: (212) 430-3333.

Project Inform Information Hotline National: (800) 822-7422; California: (800) 334-7422; San Francisco: (415) 558-9051

Clinical Trials Information Hotline, provided by the Division of AIDS, National Institute of Allergy and Infectious Diseases, National Institutes of Health. HIV-positive persons can obtain information about availability of clinical trials of medications: (800) TRIALS-A.

National Drug Information and Referral Line
National Institute of Drug Abuse. (800) 662-HELP

National Native American AIDS Prevention Center
Indian AIDS Hotline (800) 283-AIDS

In addition, more than half of the states have 800 number hotlines.

WOMEN'S ISSUES

Association for Women's Research and Education
Ward 844
San Francisco General Hospital
995 Potrero Ave.
San Francisco, CA 94110
Phone: (415) 476-4081

Haitian Women's Project
American Friends Service Committee
15 Rutherford Place
New York, NY 10003
Phone: (212) 598-0965

National Research Center on Women and AIDS
2000 P St. NW
Washington, DC 20036
Phone: (202) 872-1770

Women's AIDS Network
San Francisco AIDS Foundation
333 Valencia St.
San Francisco, CA 94101
Phone: (415) 864-4376

References

Abrams, D. I. (1990). Definition of ARC. In P. T. Cohen, M. A. Sande, & P. A. Volberding (Eds.), *The AIDS knowledge base* (pp. 4.1.3-1–4.1.3-3). Waltham, MA: Medical Publishing Group.

Adler, G., & Beckett, A. (1989). Psychotherapy of the patient with an HIV infection: Some ethical and therapeutic dilemmas. *Psychosomatics, 30,* 203–208.

Ajzen, I., & Fishbein, M. (1980). *Understanding attitudes and predicting social behavior.* Englewood Cliffs, NJ: Prentice-Hall.

Altman, L. K. (1990, June 12). Advances in treatment change face of AIDS. *New York Times.* pp. C1, C5.

American Health Consultants. (1989, June). Health care providers shun drug addicts with AIDS. *AIDS Alert, 4,* 93–102.

American Psychiatric Association. (1987). *Diagnostic and statistical manual of mental disorders* (3rd ed. rev.) Washington, DC: Author.

Annas, G. J. (1987). Protecting the liberty of pregnant patients. [Editorial]. *New England Journal of Medicine, 316,* 1213–1214.

Arno, P. S., Shenson, D., Siegel, N. F., Franks, P., & Lee, P. R. (1989). Economic and policy implications of early intervention in HIV diseases. *Journal of the American Medical Association, 262,* 1493–1498.

Ayd, F. J., Jr. (1985). Psychostimulant therapy for depressed medically ill patients. *Psychiatric Annals, 15,* 462–465.

Ayd, F. J., Jr. (1988). Psychopharmacology for HIV infected, AIDS-related complex (ARC) and AIDS patients. *International Drug Therapy Newsletter, 23,* 25–28.

Bacchetti, P., & Moss, A. R. (1989). Incubation period of AIDS in San Francisco. *Nature, 338,* 251–253.

Baer, J. W. (1989). Study of 60 patients with AIDS or AIDS-related complex requiring psychiatric hospitalization. *American Journal of Psychiatry, 146,* 1285–1288.

Baltimore, D., & Feinberg, M. B. (1989). HIV revealed. Toward a natural history of the infection. *New England Journal of Medicine, 321,* 1673–1675.

Bandura, A. (1977). *Social learning theory.* Englewood Cliffs, NJ: Prentice-Hall.

Barlow, D. H. (1988). *Anxiety and its disorders: The nature and treatment of anxiety and panic.* New York: Guilford Press.

Batki, S. L., Sorensen, J. L., Faltz, B., & Madover, S. (1988). Psychiatric aspects of treatment of IV drug abusers with AIDS. *Hospital and Community Psychiatry, 39,* 439–441.

Beck, A. T., Ward, C. H., Mendelson, M., Mock, J., & Erbaugh, J. K. (1961). An inventory for measuring depression. *Archives of General Psychiatry, 4,* 561–571.

Becker, E. (1973). *The denial of death.* New York: Free Press.

Beltangady, M. (1988). The risk of suicide in persons with AIDS [Letter to the editor]. *Journal of the American Medical Association, 260,* 29.

Benjamin, A. E. (1989). Perspectives on a continuum of care for persons with HIV illnesses. In W. N. LeVee (Ed.), *Conference proceedings. New perspectives on HIV-related illnesses: Progress in health services research* (DHHS Publication No. PHS 89-3449). Rockville, MD: National Center for Health Services Research and Health Care Technology Assessment.

Bennett, C. L., Garfinkle, J. B., Greenfield, S., Draper, D., Rogers, W., Mathews, W. C., & Kanouse, D. E. (1989). The relation between hospital experience and in-hospital mortality for patients with AIDS-related PCP. *Journal of the American Medical Association, 261,* 2975–2979.

Benton, A. L. (1968). Differential behavioral effects in frontal lobe disease. *Neuropsychologia, 6,* 53–60.

Benton, A. L. (1974). *The revised visual retention test* (4th ed). New York: Psychological Corporation.

Beral, V., Peterman, T., Berkelman, R., & Jaffe, H. (1990). Kaposi's sarcoma among persons with AIDS: A sexually transmitted infection. *Lancet, 355,* 123–128.

Berg, R., Franzen, M., & Wedding, D. (1987). *Screening for brain impairment: A manual for mental health practice.* New York: Springer.

Bialer, P. A., & Wallack, J. J. (1990). Mixed factitious disorder presenting as AIDS. *Hospital and Community Psychiatry, 41,* 552–553.

Blessed, G., Tomlinson, B. E., & Roth, M. (1968). Association between quantitative measures of dementia and of senile change in the cerebral grey matter of elderly subjects. *British Journal of Psychiatry, 114,* 797–811.

Bregman, D. J., & Langmuir, A. D. (1990). Farr's law applied to AIDS projections. *Journal of the American Medical Association, 263,* 1522–1525.

Brew, B., Rosenblum, M., & Price, R. W. (1988). Central and peripheral nervous system complications of HIV infection and AIDS. In V. T. Devita, Jr., S. Hellman, & S. A. Rosenberg (Eds.), *AIDS, etiology, diagnosis, treatment, and prevention* (2nd ed.) (pp. 185–197). Philadelphia: J. B. Lippincott.

Brooks-Gunn, J., Boyer, C. B., & Hein, K. (1988). Preventing HIV infection and AIDS in children and adolescents: Behavioral research and intervention strategies. *American Psychologist, 43,* 958–964.

Brown, V. B., Ridgely, M. S., Pepper, B., Levine, I. S., & Ryglewicz, H. (1989). The dual crisis: Mental illness and substance abuse. *American Psychologist, 44,* 565–569.

Bunis, D. (1989, November 5). AIDS in the workplace. Coping with fear of losing job, insurance. *New York Newsday,* pp. 86, 78.

Burke, D. S., Brundage, J. F., Redfield, R. R., Damato, J. J., Schable, C. A., Putman, P., Visintine, R., & Kim, H. I. (1988). Measurement of the false positive rate in a screening program for human immunodeficiency virus infections. *New England Journal of Medicine, 319,* 961–964.

Centers for Disease Control. (1987, August 14). Revision of the CDC surveillance case definition for acquired immunodeficiency syndrome. *Morbidity and Mortality Weekly Report Supplement, 36* (Suppl 1), 35–155.

Centers for Disease Control. (1989). Current trends: Coordinated community programs for HIV prevention among intravenous drug users—California, Massachusetts. *Morbidity and Mortality Weekly Report, 38,* 369–374.

Chase, M. (1989, September 15). Burroughs Wellcome reaps profits, outrage from its AIDS drug. *Wall Street Journal,* p. 1.

Citizens Commission on AIDS for New York City and Northern New Jersey. (1989). *AIDS prevention and education: Reframing the message.* New York, NY: Author.

Clark, J. M. (1986) AIDS, death, and God: Gay liberation theology and the problem of suffering. *Journal of Pastoral Counseling, 21,* 40–53.

Coates, T. J., & Greenblatt, R. M. (1990). Behavioral change using interventions at the community level. In K. K. Holmes, P.-A. Mardh, P. F. Sparling, P. J. Wiesner, W. Cates, Jr., S. M. Lemon, & W. E. Stamm (Eds.), *Sexually transmitted diseases* (2nd ed.) (pp. 1075–1080). New York: McGraw-Hill.

Coates, T. J., Stall, R., Mandel, J. S., Boccellari, A., Sorensen, J. L., Morales, E. F., Morin, S. F., Wiley, J. A., & McKusick, L. (1987). AIDS: A psychosocial research agenda. *Annals of Behavioral Medicine, 9,* 21–28.

Cochran, S. D., & Mays, V. M. (1989). Women and AIDS-related concerns. *American Psychologist, 44,* 529–535.

Cohen, P. T. (1990). Assays for HIV nucleic acid: the Polymerase Chain Reaction. In P. T. Cohen, M. A. Sande, & P. A. Volberding (Eds.), *The AIDS knowledge base* (pp. 2.1.5-1–2.1.5-5). Waltham, MA: Medical Publishing Group.

Cohen, P. T., Sande, M. A., & Volberding, P. A. (Eds.) (1990). *The AIDS knowledge base.* Waltham, MA: Medical Publishing Group.

Communication Technologies, Inc. (1987). *A report on designing an effective AIDS prevention campaign strategy for San Francisco: Results from the fourth probability sample of an urban gay male community.* Unpublished report to the San Francisco AIDS Foundation. San Francisco: Author. (Available from the San Francisco AIDS Foundation, San Francisco, CA)

Conforti, P. (1987). Reflections for Randall. Unpublished paper.

Corcoran, D. (1989, November 27). Legalizing drugs: Failures spur debate. *New York Times,* p. A15.

Cotton, P. (1990). Controversy continues as experts ponder zidovudine's role in early HIV infection. *Journal of the American Medical Association, 263,* 1605.

Crewdson, J. (1989, November 19). The great AIDS quest. *Chicago Tribune,* Sec. 5, pp. 1–16.

Crewdson, J. (1990, March 18). Inquiry hid facts on AIDS research. *Chicago Tribune,* pp. 1, 16–17.

Crowe, S. M., & McGrath, M. S. (1990). Acute HIV infection. In P. T. Cohen, M. A. Sande, & P. A. Volberding (Eds.), *The AIDS knowledge base* (pp. 4.1.2-1–4.1.2.-4). Waltham, MA: Medical Publishing Group.

Cumming, P. D., Wallace, E. L., Schorr, J. B., & Dodd, R. Y. (1989). Exposure of patients to human immunodeficiency virus through the transfusion of blood components that test antibody-negative. *New England Journal of Medicine, 321,* 941–946.

Day, S. (1988). Prostitute women and AIDS: Anthropology. *AIDS, 2,* 429–432.

DeNoon, D. J. (Ed.). (1989, May 8). Directory of antiviral and immunomodulatory therapies for AIDS. CDC AIDS Weekly. Atlanta: CDC AIDS Weekly.

Derogatis, L. R., & Melisaratos, N. (1983). The brief symptom inventory: An introductory report. *Psychological Medicine, 13,* 595–605.

Des Jarlais, D. C., & Friedman, S. R. (1988). The psychology of preventing AIDS among intravenous drug users: A social learning conceptualization. *American Psychologist, 43,* 865–870.

Des Jarlais, D. C., Friedman, S. R., Novick, D. M., Sotheran, J. L., Thomas, P.,

Yancovitz, S. R., Mildvan, D., Weber, J., Kreek, M. J., Maslansky, R., Bartelme, S., Spira, T., & Marmor, M. (1989). HIV-1 infection among intravenous drug users in Manhattan, New York City, from 1977 through 1987. *Journal of the American Medical Association, 261,* 1008–1012.

Diesenhouse, S. (1990, January 7). Drug treatment is scarcer than ever for women. *New York Times,* Sec. 4, p. 26.

Doll, L., Darrow, W. W., Jaffe, H., Curran, L., O'Malley, P., Bodecker, T., Campbel, J., & Franks, D. (1987, June). *Self-reported changes in sexual behaviors in gay and bisexual men from the San Francisco City Clinic Cohort.* Paper presented at the Third International Conference on AIDS, Washington, DC.

Douglas, C. J., Kalman, C. M., & Kalman, T. (1985). Homophobia among physicians and nurses: An empirical study. *Hospital and Community Psychiatry, 36,* 1309–1311.

Dunn, L. M., & Dunn, L. M. (1981). *Peabody Picture Vocabulary Test—Revised Manual.* Circle Pines, MN: American Guidance Service.

Elder, G. A., & Sever, J. L. (1988). Neurological disorders associated with AIDS retroviral infection. *Reviews of Infectious Diseases, 10,* 286–295.

Essex, M. & Kanki, P. J. (1988, October). The origins of the AIDS virus. *Scientific American, 259,* 64–71.

Faltz, B., & Madover, S. (1987). Co-dependency in AIDS: A clinical perspective. In P. L. Petrakis (Ed.), *Acquired immune deficiency syndrome and chemical dependency: Report of a symposium sponsored by the American Medical Society on Alcoholism and Other Drug Dependencies and the National Council on Alcoholism* (pp. 61–66) (DHHS Publication No. ADM 87-1513). Washington, DC: U.S. Government Printing Office.

Faltz, B., & Rinaldi, J. (1988). *AIDS and substance abuse.* San Francisco: University of California AIDS Health Project.

Fernandez, F., Adams, F., Levy, J. K., Holmes, V. F., Neidhart, M., & Mansell, P. W. A. (1988). Cognitive impairment due to AIDS-related complex and its response to psychostimulants. *Psychosomatics, 29,* 38–45.

Fernandez, F., Levy, J. K., & Galizz, H. (1988). Response of HIV-related depression to psychostimulants: Case reports. *Hospital and Community Psychiatry, 39,* 628–631.

Fischl, M. A., Richman, D. D., Hansen, N., Collier, A. C., Carey, J. T., Para, M. F., Hardy, W. D., Dolin, R., Powderly, W. G., Allan, J. D., Wong, B., Merigan, T. C., McAuliffe, V. J., Hyslop, N. E., Rhame, F. S., Balfour, H. H., Jr., Spector, S. A., Volberding, P., Pettinelli, C., Anderson, J., & the AIDS Clinical Trials Group. (1990). Safety and efficacy of zidovudine (AZT) in the treatment of subjects with mildly symptomatic human immunodeficiency virus type 1 (HIV) infection. A double-blind, placebo-controlled trial. *Annals of Internal Medicine, 112,* 727–737.

Flora, J. A., & Thoresen, C. E. (1988). Reducing the risk of AIDS in adolescents. *American Psychologist, 43,* 971–976.

Fowles, D. C. (1988). Models of addiction [Special issue]. *Journal of Abnormal Psychology, 97* (2).

Friedland, G. (1990). Early treatment for HIV. The time has come [Editorial]. *New England Journal of Medicine, 322,* 1000–1002.

Friedland, G. H., & Klein, R. S. (1987). Transmission of the human immunodeficiency virus. *New England Journal of Medicine, 317,* 1125–1135.

Frierson, R. L., & Lippmann, S. B. (1988). Suicide and AIDS. *Psychosomatics, 29,* 226–231.

Fullilove, R. E., Fullilove, M. T., Bowser, B. P., & Gross, S. A. (1990). Risk of sexually transmitted disease among black adolescent crack users in Oakland and San Francisco, California. *Journal of the American Medical Association, 263,* 851–855.

Gail, M. H., & Brookmeyer, R. (1990). Projecting the incidence of AIDS [Editorial]. *Journal of the American Medical Association, 263,* 1538–1539.

Gelberding, J. (1990, June). Chemoprophylaxis for occupational exposure. Symposium conducted at the Sixth International Conference on AIDS. San Francisco, CA.

Goedert, J. J., Kessler, C. M., Aledort, L. M., Biggar, R. J., Andes, W. A., White, G. C., II, Drummond, J. E., Vaidya, K., Mann, D. L., Eyster, M. E., Ragni, M. V., Lederman, M. M., Cohen, A. R., Bray, G. L., Rosenberg, P. S., Friedman, R. M., Hilgartner, M. W., Blattner, W. A., Kroner, B., & Gail, M. H. (1989). A prospective study of human immunodeficiency virus type 1 infection and the development of AIDS in subjects with hemophilia. *New England Journal of Medicine, 321,* 1141–1148.

Gold, A. R. (1989, August 1). Fodor is freed without bail in drug case. *New York Times,* p. C14.

Goldberg, R. J. (1987). The assessment of suicide risk in the general hospital. *General Hospital Psychiatry, 9,* 446–452.

Green, L. W., Reuter, M. W., Deeds, S., & Partridge, K. B. (1980). *Health education planning: A diagnostic approach.* Palo Alto, CA: Mayfield.

Groves, J. E., & Vaccarino, J. M. (1987). In T. P. Hackett & N. H. Cassem (Eds.), *Massachusetts General Hospital handbook of general hospital psychiatry* (pp. 591–617). Littleton, MA: PSG.

Hahn, B. H., Gonda, M. A., Shaw, G. M., Popovic, M., Hoxie, J., Gallo, R. C., & Wong-Staal, F. (1985). Genomic diversity of the AIDS virus HTLV-III: Different viruses exhibit greatest divergence in their envelope genes. *Proceedings of the National Academy of Sciences, USA, 82,* 4813–4817.

Haislip, G. R. (1989, August 2). Statement of Gene R. Haislip, deputy assistant administrator, office of diversion control, Drug Enforcement Administration, on methadone diversion from narcotic treatment programs to the Select Committee on Narcotics Abuse and Control.

Hall, N. R. S. (1988). Virology of AIDS. *American Psychologist, 43,* 907–913.

Halstead, W. C. (1947). *Brain and intelligence.* Chicago: University of Chicago Press.

Harris, J. E. (1990). Improved short-term survival of AIDS patients initially diagnosed with *pneumocystis carinii* pneumonia, 1984–1987. *Journal of the American Medical Association, 263,* 397–401.

Hearst, N., & Hulley, S. B. (1988). Preventing the heterosexual spread of AIDS. Are we giving our patients the best advice? *Journal of the American Medical Association, 259,* 2428–2432.

Hirsch, V. M., Omsted, R. A., Murphey-Corb, M., Purcell, R. H., & Johnson, P. R. (1989). An African primate lentivirus closely related to HIV-2. *Nature, 339,* 389–391.

Ho, D. D., Pomerantz, R. J., & Kaplan, J. C. (1987). Pathogenesis of infection with human immunodeficiency virus. *New England Journal of Medicine, 317,* 278–286.

Hoban, P. (1989, December 4). Prodigal son. After the drug bust, Eugene Fodor tries a comeback. *New York Times,* pp. 100–116.

Holland, J. C., & Tross, S. (1985). The psychosocial and neuropsychiatric sequalae of the acquired immune deficiency syndrome and related disorders. *Annals of Internal Medicine, 103,* 760–764.

Holmes, V., Fernandez, F., & Levy, J. K. (1989). Psychostimulant response in AIDS-related complex (ARC) patients. *Journal of Clinical Psychiatry, 50,* 5–8.

Holmes, V., & Fricchione, G. L. (1989). Hypomania in an AIDS patient receiving amitriptyline for neuropathic pain. *Neurology, 39,* 305.

Hull, H. F., Sewell, C. M., Wilson, J., & McFeeley, P. (1988). The risk of suicide in persons with AIDS [Letter to the editor]. *Journal of the American Medical Association, 260,* 29–30.

Institute of Medicine/National Academy of Sciences. (1988). *Confronting AIDS: Update 1988.* Washington, DC: National Academy Press.

Jackson, J., & Rotkiewicz, L. (1987, June). *A coupon program: AIDS education and drug treatment.* Paper presented at the Third International Conference on AIDS, Washington, DC.

Johnston, W. B., & Hopkins, K. R. (1989). *The catastrophe ahead: AIDS and the case for a new public policy.* Indianapolis, IN: Hudson Institute.

Justice, A. C., Feinstein, A. R., & Wells, C. K. (1989). A new prognostic staging system for the Acquired Immunodeficiency Syndrome. *New England Journal of Medicine, 320,* 1388–1393.

Kaemingk, K. L., & Kaszniak, A. W. (1989). Neuropsychological aspects of human immunodeficiency virus infection. *Clinical Neuropsychologist, 3,* 309–326.

Kelly, J. A., & St. Lawrence, J. S. (1988). AIDS prevention and treatment: Psychology's role in the health crisis. *Clinical Psychology Review, 8,* 255–284.

Kelly, J. A., & St. Lawrence, J. S. (1990). *Behavioral group intervention to teach AIDS risk reduction skills.* Jackson, MS: University of Mississippi Medical Center.

Kelly, J. A., St. Lawrence, J. S., Hood, H. V., & Brasfield, T. L. (1989). Behavioral intervention to reduce AIDS risk activities. *Journal of Consulting and Clinical Psychology, 57,* 60–67.

Kernberg, O. F. (1984). *Severe personality disorders.* New Haven, CT: Yale University Press.

Kerr, P. (1989, August 20). Crack and resurgence of syphilis spreading AIDS among the poor. *New York Times,* pp. 1, 36.

Khantzian, E. J. (1985). The self-medication hypothesis of addictive disorders: Focus on heroin and cocaine dependence. *American Journal of Psychiatry, 142,* 1259–1264.

Khantzian, E. J., Mack, J. E., & Schatzberg, A. F. (1974). Heroin use as an attempt to cope: Clinical observations. *American Journal of Psychiatry, 131,* 160–164.

Kizer, K. W., Green, M., Perkins, C. I., Doebbert, G., & Hughes, M. J. (1988). AIDS and suicide in California [Letter to the editor]. *Journal of the American Medical Association, 260,* 1881.

Klove, H. (1963). Clinical neuropsychology. In F. M. Forster (Ed.), *Medical clinics of North America.* New York: Saunders.

Kolata, G. (1989, December 24). AIDS strategy for addicts is faulted. *New York Times,* p. 19.

Kolata, G. (1990, March 9). Trial of experimental AIDS drug to be continued, with revisions. *New York Times,* pp. 1, A15.

Kolder, V. E. B., Gallagher, J., & Parsons, M. T. (1987). Court-ordered obstetrical interventions. *New England Journal of Medicine, 316,* 1192–1196.

Kreek, M. J. (1983). Factors modifying the pharmacological effectiveness of methadone. In J. R. Cooper, F. Altman, B. S. Brown, & D. Czechowicz (Eds.), *Research in treatment of narcotic addiction* (pp. 95–107) (DHHS Publication No. ADM 83–1281). Treatment Research Monograph Series. Washington: Department of Health and Human Services.

Kreek, M. J., Garfield, J. W., Gutjarh, C. L., & Guisti, I. M. (1976). Rifampin-induced methadone withdrawal. *New England Journal of Medicine, 294,* 1104–1106.

Kübler-Ross, E. (1969). *On death and dying.* New York: Macmillan.

Kuhn, T. S. (1970). *The structure of scientific revolutions.* Chicago, IL: University of Chicago Press.

Kushner, H. S. (1981). *When bad things happen to good people.* New York: Avon.

Lambert, B. (1989, November 15) Health board backs move to trace AIDS. Joseph still seeks to list drug and sex partners. *New York Times,* pp. B1, B10.

Lancet (1990). Zidovudine for symptomless HIV infection [Editorial]. *Lancet, 335,* 821–822.

Lapham, L. H. (1989, December). A political opiate. The war on drugs is a folly and a menace. *Harper's,* pp. 43–48.

Lemp, G. F., Payne, S. F., Neal, D., Temelso, T., & Rutherford, G. W. (1990). Survival trends for patients with AIDS. *Journal of the American Medical Association, 263,* 402–406.

LeVee, W. N. (1989). *Conference proceedings. New perspectives on HIV-related illnesses: Progress in health services research* (DHHS Publication No. PHS 89-3449). Rockville, MD: National Center for Health Services Research and Health Care Technology Assessment.

Levine, S. (1984). *Meetings at the edge.* New York: Anchor Books.

Levy, J. A. (1990, June). *Changing concepts in HIV infection: Challenges for the 1990s.* Paper presented at the Sixth International Conference on AIDS. San Francisco, CA.

Levy, R. M., & Bredesen, D. E. (1988). Central nervous system dysfunction is acquired immunodeficiency syndrome. *Journal of Acquired Immune Deficiency Syndromes, 1,* 41–64.

Levy, R. M., Bredesen, D. E., & Rosenblum, M. L. (1988). Opportunistic central nervous system pathology in patients with AIDS. *Annals of Neurology, 23* (Suppl), S7–S16.

Lewis, H. B. (1971). *Shame and guilt in neurosis.* New York: International Universities Press.

Lezak, M. D. (1983). *Neuropsychological assessment (2nd ed.).* New York: Oxford University Press.

Lifson, A., Hessol, N., Rutherford, G. W., Buchbinder, S., O'Malley, P., Cannon, L., Barnhart, L., Harrison, J., Doll, L., Holmberg, S., & Jaffe, H. (1989, June). Natural history of HIV infection in a cohort of homosexual and bisexual men: Clinical manifestations, 1978–1989. *Proceedings and abstracts of the Fifth International Conference on AIDS,* Montreal, Canada.

Lindsay-Hartz, J. (1984). Contrasting experiences of shame and guilt. *American Behavioral Scientist, 27,* 689–704.

Linn, L. S., Spiegel, J. S., Mathews, W. C., Leake, B., Lien, R., & Brooks, S. (1989). Recent sexual behaviors among homosexual men seeking primary medical care. *Archives of Internal Medicine, 149,* 2685–2690.

Lo, S.-Y., Shih, J. W.-K., Newton, P. B., III, Wong, D. M., Hayes, M. M., Benish, J. R., Wear, D. J., & Wang, R. Y.-H. (1989). Virus-like infectious agent (VLIA) in a novel pathogenic mycoplasma: Mycoplasma incognitus. *American Journal of Tropical Medicine and Hygiene, 41,* 586–600.

Lo, S.-Y., Shih, J. W.-K., Yang, N.-Y., Ou, C.-Y., & Wang, R. Y.-H. (1989). A novel virus-like infectious agent in patients with AIDS. *American Journal of Tropical Medicine and Hygiene, 40,* 213–226.

MacDonald, K. L., Jackson, J. B., Bowman, R. J., Polesky, H. F., Rhame, F. S., Balfour, H. H., Jr., & Osterholm, M. T. (1989). Performance characteristics of serologic tests for human immunodeficiency virus type 1 (HIV-1) antibody among Minnesota blood donors. Public health and clinical implications. *Annals of Internal Medicine, 110,* 617–621.

Malow, R. M., West, J. A., Williams, J. L., & Sutker, P. B. (1989). Personality disorders classification and symptoms in cocaine and opioid addicts. *Journal of Consulting and Clinical Psychology, 57,* 765–767.

Mann, J. M. (1989). Global AIDS into the 1990s. (Publication GPA/DIR/89.2, English). Geneva: World Health Organization

Marlatt, G. A., & Gordon, J. R. (Eds.). (1985). *Relapse prevention: Maintenance strategies in the treatment of addiction.* New York: Guilford.

Marmor, M., Weiss, L. R., Lyden, M., Weiss, S. H., Saxinger, W. C., Spira, T. J., & Feorino, P. M. (1986). Possible female-to-female transmission of human immunodeficiency virus [Letter]. *Annals of Internal Medicine, 105,* 969.

Martin, J. L. (1988). Psychological consequences of AIDS-related bereavement among gay men. *Journal of Consulting and Clinical Psychology, 56,* 856–862.

Martin, J. L. (1990). Drug use and unprotected anal intercourse among gay men. *Health Psychology, 9,* 450–465.

Marzuk, P. M., Tierney, H., Tardiff, K., Gross, E. M., Morgan, E. B., Hsu, M.-A., & Mann, J. J. (1988). Increased risk of suicide in persons with AIDS. *Journal of the American Medical Association, 259,* 1333–1337.

Matarazzo, J. D., & Herman, D. O. (1984). Relationship of education and IQ in the WAIS-R standardization sample. *Journal of Consulting and Clinical Psychology, 52,* 631–634.

Mays, V. M., & Cochran, S. D. (1988). Issues in the perception of AIDS risk and risk reduction activities by black and Hispanic/Latina women. *American Psychologist, 43,* 949–957.

McArthur, J. C. (1987). Neurologic manifestations of AIDS. *Medicine, 66,* 407–437.

McAuliffe, W. E., Doering, S., Breer, P., Silverman, H., Branson, B., & Williams, K. (1987, June). *An evaluation of using ex-addict outreach workers to educate intravenous drug users about AIDS prevention.* Paper presented at the Third International Conference on AIDS, Washington, DC.

McKusick, L. (1988). Impact of AIDS on practitioner and client. *American Psychologist, 43,* 935–940.

Meichenbaum, D. (1985). *Stress inoculation training.* Elmsford, NY: Pergamon Press.

Melton, J. G. (1989). *The churches speak on: AIDS.* Detroit, MI: Gale Research.

Miller, I. W., Norman, W. H., & Keitner, G. I. (1989). Cognitive-behavioral treatment of depressed inpatients: Six- and twelve-month follow-up. *American Journal of Psychiatry, 146,* 1274–1279.

Miller, E. N., Selnes, O. A., McArthur, J. C., Satz, P., Becker, J. T., Cohen, M. D., Sheridan, K., Machado, A. M., Van Gorp., W. G., & Visscher, B. (1990). Neuropsychological performance in HIV-1-infected homosexual men: The multicenter AIDS cohort study (MACS). *Neurology, 40,* 197–203.

Montagnier, L. (1990, June). *HIV pathogenesis.* Paper presented at the Sixth International Conference on AIDS. San Francisco, CA.

Moorhead, C. (1989, July). *Parallel processing: Persons with AIDS and their caregivers.* Paper presented at the National Catholic AIDS Ministry Conference, South Bend, IN.

Morgan, M., Curran, J. W., & Berkelman, R. L. (1990). The future course of AIDS in the United States [Editorial]. *Journal of the American Medical Association, 263,* 1539–1540.

Mueller, J. (1984). Mental status examination. In H. H. Goldman (Ed.), *Review of general psychiatry.* Los Altos, CA: Lange Medical.

National Commission on Acquired Immune Deficiency Syndrome. (1989, December 5). Report number one. Washington, DC: Author.

National Institute of Allergy and Infectious Diseases. (1989a, August 29). Results of controlled clinical trials of ziovudine in early HIV infection. *AIDS Clinical Trials Alert.* Washington, DC: Author.

National Institute of Allergy and Infectious Diseases. (1989b). *AIDS clinical trials. Talking it over.* (NIH Publication No. 89-3025). Washington, DC: Author.

National Institute of Allergy and Infectious Diseases (NIAID). (1990). Recommendations for zidovudine. Early infection. *Journal of the American Medical Association, 263,* 1606–1609.

Navia, B. A., Cho, E. S., Petito, C. K., & Price, R. W. (1986). The AIDS dementia complex II. Neuropathology. *Annals of Neurology, 19,* 525–535.

Navia, B. A., Jordan, B. D., & Price, R. W. (1986). AIDS dementia complex: I. Clinical features. *Annals of Neurology, 19,* 517–524.

New York City Department of Health. (1987). *AIDS and drugs.* (No. A1003). New York: Author.

New York City Department of Health. (1989). *The pilot needle exchange study in New York City: A bridge to treatment.* New York: Author.

North, R. L., & Rothenberg, K. H. (1990). The duty to warn "dilemma:" A framework for resolution. *AIDS & Public Policy Journal, 4,* 133–141.

Osmond, D. (1990). AIDS in Africa. In P. T. Cohen, M. A. Sande, & P. A. Volberding (Eds.), *The AIDS knowledge base* (pp. 1.1.4-1–1.1.4-10). Waltham, MA: Medical Publishing Group.

Padian, N. S. (1988). Prostitute women and AIDS: Epidemiology. *AIDS, 2,* 421–428.

Padian, N. S., & Francis, D. P. (1988). Preventing the heterosexual spread of AIDS [Letter to the editor]. *Journal of the American Medical Association, 260,* 1879.

Perry, S. W. (1990). Organic mental disorders caused by HIV: Update on early diagnosis and treatment. *American Journal of Psychiatry, 147,* 696–710.

Perry, S., Jacobsberg, L., & Fishman, B. (1990). Suicidal ideation and HIV testing. *Journal of the American Medical Association, 263,* 679–682.

Perry, S., Jacobsberg, L. B., Fishman, B., Frances, A., Bobo, J., & Jacobsberg, B. K. (1990). Psychiatric diagnosis before serological testing for the human immunodeficiency virus. *American Journal of Psychiatry, 147,* 89–93.

Peterson, J. L., & Marin, G. (1988). Issues in the prevention of AIDS among black and hispanic men. *American Psychologist, 43,* 871–877.

Phair, J., Munoz, A., Detels, R., Kaslow, R., Rinaldo, C., Saah, A., and the Multicenter AIDS Cohort Study Group. (1990). Risk of *pneumocystis carinii* pneumonia among men infected with human immunodeficiency virus type 1. *New England Journal of Medicine, 322,* 161–165.

Pitta, A. (1990, February). Tuberculosis and other mycobacteria. Presentation at Spellman Center for HIV-Related Disease, New York, NY.

Pollack, B. (1942). The validity of the Shipley–Hartford Retreat Test for "deterioration." *Psychiatric Quarterly, 16,* 119–131.

Presidential Commission on the Human Immunodeficiency Virus Epidemic. (1988). *Report of the Presidential Commission on the Human Immunodeficiency Virus.* (1988 0-214-701:QL3) Washington, DC: U.S. Government Printing Office.

Price, R. W., & Brew, B. (1988). Management of the neurological complications of HIV infection and AIDS. In M. A. Sande, & P. A. Volberding (Eds.), *Medical management of AIDS* (pp. 111–126). Philadelphia: W. B. Saunders.

Price, R. W., Brew, B., Sidtis, J., Rosenblum, M., Scheck, A. C., & Cleary, P. (1988). The brain in AIDS: Central nervous system HIV-1 infection and AIDS dementia complex. *Science, 239,* 586–592.

Rapoport, J. L. (1990). *The boy who couldn't stop washing.* New York: Plume.

Ratner, L., Gallo, R. C., & Wong-Staal, F. (1985). HTLV-III, LAV and ARV are variants of the same AIDS virus. *Nature, 313,* 636–637.

Raven, J. C. (n.d.). *Guide to the Standard Progressive Matrices.* New York: Psychological Corporation.

Redfield, R. R., Markham, P. D., Salahuddin, S. Z., Wright, D. C., Sarngadharan, M. G., & Gallo, R. C. (1985). Heterosexually acquired HTLV-III/LAV disease (AIDS-related complex and AIDS): Epidemiologic evidence for female-to-male transmission. *Journal of the American Medical Association, 254,* 2094–2096.

Redfield, R. R., Wright, D. D., & Tramont, E. C. (1986). The Walter Reed staging classification for HTLV-III/LAV infection. *New England Journal of Medicine, 314,* 131–132.

Reitan, R. M. (1979). *Manual for administration of neuropsychological test batteries for adults and children.* Tucson: Reitan Neuropsychology Laboratories.

Rey, A. (1964). *L'examen clinique en psychologie* [The clinical examination in psychology]. Paris: Presses Universitaires de France.

Rook, A. H., Hooks, J. J., Quinnan, G. V., Lane, H. C., Manischewitz, J. F., Jackson, L., Fauci, A. S., & Quinnan, G. V., Jr. (1985). Interleukin-2 enhances the natural killer cell activity of acquired immunodeficiency syndrome patients through a *g* interferon-independent mechanism. *Journal of Immunology, 134,* 1503–1507.

Rosenbaum, J. F., & Pollack, M. H. (1987). Anxiety. In T. P. Hackett & N. H. Cassem (Eds.), *Massachusetts General Hospital handbook of general hospital psychiatry* (2nd ed., pp. 154–183). Littleton, MA: PSG.

Ross, H. E., Glaser, F. B., & Germanson, T. (1988). The prevalence of psychiatric disorders in patients with alcohol and other drug problems. *Archives of General Psychiatry, 45,* 1023–1031.

Ruben, D. S., Eagan, J. A., Burns, J. M., Berger, B. J., Taneja-Uppal, N., Urban, C. M., & Rahal, J. J. (1989, September). Risk denial among HIV-infected males in a middle-class urban community. Presentation at the 29th Interscience Conference on Antimicrobial Agents and Chemotherapy, Houston, TX.

Ruedy, J., Schechter, M., & Montaner, J. S. G. (1990). Zidovudine for early human immunodeficiency virus (HIV) infection: Who, when, and how? *Annals of Internal Medicine, 112,* 721–723.

Salzman, C. (1990, March). What are the uses and dangers of the controversial drug, Halcion? *Harvard Medical School Mental Health Letter, 6,* 8.

Schneidman, E. S. (1983). *Deaths of man.* New York: Jason Aronson.

Schoenbaum, E. E., Hartel, D., Selwyn, P. A., Klein, R. S., Davenny, K., Rogers, M., Feiner, C., & Friedland, G. (1989). Risk factors for human immuodeficiency virus infection in intravenous drug users. *New England Journal of Medicine, 321,* 874–879.

Selnes, O. A., Miller, E., McArthur, J., Gordon, B., Munoz, A., Sheridan, K., Fox, R., Saah, A. J., and the Multicenter AIDS Cohort Study Group. (1990). HIV-1 infection: No evidence of cognitive decline during the asymptomatic stages. *Neurology, 40,* 204–208.

Selwyn, P. A. (1989). Issues in the clinical management of intravenous drug users with HIV infection. *AIDS, 3* (Suppl 1), S201–S208.

Seravalli, E. P. (1988). The dying patient, the physician, and the fear of death. *New England Journal of Medicine, 319,* 1728–1730.

Sestak, P., Schechter, M. T., Willoughby, B., Craib, K. J. P., Maynard, M., O'Shaughnessy, M. V., Nitz, R., Le, T. N., Broughton, S., & Fay, S. (1989, June). Incidence of seroconversion and risk factors in a cohort of homosexual men: Results at six years. Presentation at the Fifth International Conference on AIDS, Montreal, Canada.

Shaw, G. M., Hahn, B. H., Arya, S. K., Groopman, J. E., Gallo, R. C., & Wong-Staal, F. (1984). Molecular characterization of human T-cell leukemia (lymphotropic) virus type III in the acquired immunodeficiency syndrome. *Science, 226,* 1165–1171.

Shaw, G. M., Harper, M. E., Hahn, B. H., Epstein, L. G., Gajdusek, D. C., Price, R. W., Navia, B. A., Petito, C. K., O'Hara, C. J., Groopman, J. E., Cho, E.-S., Oleske, J. M., Wong-Staal, F., & Gallo, R. C. (1985). HTLV-III infection in brains of children and adults with AIDS encephalopathy. *Science, 227,* 177–182.

Shikles, J. L. (1989, August 2). Preliminary findings: A survey of methadone maintenance programs. U.S. General Accounting Office statement to the House Select Committee on Narcotics Abuse and Control, House of Representatives.

Shilts, R. (1988). *And the band played on.* New York: Penguin.

Sidtis, J. J., & Price R. W. (1990). Early HIV-1 infection and the AIDS dementia complex [Editorial]. *Neurology, 40,* 323–326.

Smith, A. (1982). *Symbol digits modalities test.* Los Angeles: Western Psychological Services.

Sparrow, S. S., Balla, D. A., & Cicchetti, D. (1985). *Vineland Adaptive Behavioral Scales.* Circle Pines, MN: American Guidance Service, Inc.

Spitzer, P. G., & Weiner, N. J. (1989). Transmission of HIV infection from a woman to a man by oral sex [Letter]. *New England Journal of Medicine, 320,* 251.

Staff. (1989, July 24). London: Nonoxynol-9 and nonoxynol-11 are both active against HIV. *CDC AIDS Weekly,* p. 16.

Staff. (1989, November). Compound Q—The real story. *PI Perspective.* San Francisco: Project Inform.

Stall, R. D., Coates, T. J., & Hoff, C. (1988). Behavioral risk reduction for HIV infection among gay and bisexual men: A review of results from the United States. *American Psychologist, 43,* 878–885.

Stall, R., Wiley, J. A., McKusick, L., Coates, T. J., & Ostrow, D. (1986). Alcohol and drug use during sexual activity and compliance with safe sex guidelines for AIDS: The AIDS Behavioral Research Project. *Health Education Quarterly, 13,* 359–371.

Steinfels, P. (1989, November 19). Judgement is mostly compassionate. AIDS provokes theological second thoughts. *New York Times,* p. 5.

Stevens, L. A., & Muskin, P. R. (1987). Techniques for reversing the failure of empathy towards AIDS patients. *Journal of the American Academy of Psychoanalysis, 15,* 539–551.

Tangney, J. P. (1988, August). Proneness to shame, proneness to guilt, and empathic responsiveness. Presentation at the annual meeting of the American Psychological Association, Atlanta, GA.

Tarasoff v. Regents of University of California, 131 Cal. Rptr. 14, 551 P.2nd 334 (1976).

Tillich, P. (1952). *The courage to be.* New Haven: Yale University Press.

Tong, T. G., Pond, S. M., Kreek, M. J., Jaffery, N. F., & Benowitz, N. L. (1981). Phenytoin induced methadone withdrawal. *Annals of Internal Medicine, 94,* 349–351.

Trahan, D. E., Patterson, J., Quintana, J., & Biron, R. (1987). The finger tapping test: a reexamination of traditional hypotheses regarding normal adult performance [Abstract]. *Journal of Clinical and Experimental Neuropsychology, 9,* 52.

Trites, R. L. (1977). *Neuropsychological test manual.* Lafayette: Lafayette Instrument.

Tross, S., Price, R. W., Navia, B., Thaler, H. T., Gold, J., Hirsch, D. A., & Sidtis, J. J. (1988). Neuropsychological characterization of the AIDS dementia complex: A preliminary report. *AIDS, 2,* 81–88.

Tunnell, G. (1987, December). Counseling AIDS patients and their families. Presentation at Queens College, Flushing, New York.

Turner, B. J., Kelly, J. V., & Ball, J. K. (1989). A severity classification system for AIDS hospitalizations. *Medical Care, 27,* 423–437.

Vaillant, G. E. (1975). Sociopathy as a human process: A viewpoint. *Archives of General Psychiatry, 32,* 178–183.

Vogt, M. W., Witt, D. J., Craven, D. E., Byington, R., Crawford, D. F., Hutchinson, M. S., Schooley, R. T., & Hirsch, M. S. (1987). Isolation patterns of the human immunodeficiency virus from cervical secretions during the menstrual cycle of women at risk for the acquired immunodeficiency syndrome. *Annals of Internal Medicine, 106,* 380–382.

Volberding, P. A. & Cohen, P. T. (1990). Clinical spectrum of HIV infection. In P. T. Cohen, M. A. Sande, & P. A. Volberding (Eds.), *The AIDS knowledge base* (pp. 4.1.1-1–4.1.1-11). Waltham, MA: Medical Publishing Group.

Volberding, P. A., Lagakos, S. W., Koch, M. A., Pettinelli, C., Myers, M. W., Booth, D. K., Balfour, H. H., Jr., Reichman, R. C., Bartlett, J. A., Hirsch, M. S., Murphy, R. L., Hardy, W. D., Soeiro, R., Fischl, M. A., Bartlett, J. G., Merigan, T. C., Hyslop, N. E., Richman, D. D., Valentine, F. T., Corey, L., & the AIDS Clinical Trials Group of the National Institute of Allergy and Infectious Diseases. (1990). Zidovudine in asymptomatic human immunodeficiency virus infection. A controlled trial in persons with fewer than 500 CD4-positive cells per cubic millimeter. *New England Journal of Medicine, 322,* 941–949.

Wade, B. (1989, August 13). AIDS-test rules in 29 countries. *New York Times,* Travel Section, pp. 3, 26.

Wallace, R. (1988). A synergism of plagues: "Planned shrinkage," contagious housing destruction, and AIDS in the Bronx. *Environmental Research, 47,* 1–33.

Watters, J. K., Cheng, Y., Segal, M., Lorvick, J., Case, P., & Carlson, J. (1990, June). Epidemiology and prevention of HIV in intravenous drug users in San Francisco. In P. Phanuphak, & P. M. Mannucci (Chairs), *Issues in parenterally transmitted HIV infection.* Symposium conducted at the Sixth International Conference on AIDS, San Francisco, CA.

Wechsler, D. (1981). *WAIS-R manual.* New York: Psychological Corporation.

Weisman, A. D. (1981). Understanding the cancer patient: The syndrome of caregiver's plight. *Psychiatry, 44,* 161–168.

When caring for persons with AIDS—We must examine our own prejudices. (1987, November 1). *Catholic Health World,* p. 1.

Wilber, J. C. (1990). HIV antibody testing: Methodology. In P. T. Cohen, M. A. Sande, & P. A. Volberding (Eds.), *The AIDS knowledge base* (pp. 2.1.2-1–2.1.2.-8). Waltham, MA: Medical Publishing Group.

Winiarski, M. G., & Hoffman, X. (1990, June). Beck Depression Inventory and an analog scale as screening devices for hospitalized AIDS patients. Paper presented at the Sixth International Conference on AIDS, San Francisco, CA.

Wofsy, C. B., Cohen, J. B., Hauer, L. B., Padian, N. S., Michaelis, B. A., Evans, L. A., & Levy, J. A. (1986). Isolation of AIDS-associated retrovirus from genital secretions of women with antibodies to the virus. *Lancet, 1,* 527–529.

Wong-Staal, F., Shaw, G. M., Hahn, B. H., Salahuddin, S. Z., Popovic, M., Markham, P. D., Redfield, R., & Gallo R. C. (1987). Genomic diversity of human T-lymphotropic virus type III (HTLV-III). *Science, 229,* 759–762.

Woodcock, R. W., & Johnson, M. B. (1989). *Woodcock–Johnson Psycho-Educational Battery—Revised.* Allen, TX: DLM Teaching Resources.

World Health Organization. (1988). *Report of the consultation on the neuropsychiatric aspects of HIV infection.* Geneva: Author.

Wormser, G. P., & Joline, C. (1989). Would you eat cookies prepared by an AIDS patient? *Postgraduate Medicine, 86,* 174–186.

Yalom, I. D. (1980). *Existential psychotherapy.* New York: Basic Books.

Zuger, A., & Steigbigel, N. H. (1990, March/April). Heterosexual transmission of human immunodeficiency virus infection. *AIDS Updates, 3,* 1.

Author Index

Abrams, D. I., 18
Adams, F., 74
Adler, G., 50
AIDS Clinical Trials Group of NIAID, 149
Ajzen, I., 158
Aledort, L. M., 16, 18
Altman, L. K., 9
American Foundation for AIDS Research, 194
American Health Consultants, 174
American Psychiatric Association, 71, 178, 181
Anderson, J., 149
Andes, W. A., 16, 18
Annas, G. J., 35
Arno, P. S., 149
Arya, S. K., 14
Ayd, F. J., Jr., 74, 75, 76

Bacchetti, P., 18
Baer, J. W., 72, 76, 89–90
Balfour, H. H., Jr., 17, 149
Ball, J. K., 20
Balla, D. A., 95
Baltimore, D., 17
Bandura, A., 158

Barlow, D. H., 75
Barnhart, L., 18
Bartelme, S., 159
Bartlett, J. A., 149
Bartlett, J. G., 149
Batki, S. L., 113, 166, 170, 172
Beck, A. T., 73
Becker, E., 31, 130
Becker, J. T., 84–85, 91, 92
Beckett, A., 50
Beltangady, M., 78
Benish, J. R., 87
Benjamin, A. E., 98
Bennett, C. L., 33, 44
Benowitz, N. L., 176
Benton, A. L., 91, 92
Beral, V., 8
Berg, R., 45, 71
Berger, B. J., 16
Berkelman, R. L., 8, 9
Bialer, P. A., 182
Biggar, R. J., 16, 18
Biron, R., 91
Blattner, W. A., 16, 18
Blessed, G., 46
Bobo, J., 73
Boccellari, A., 156

221

Subject Index

About the Author

Mark G. Winiarski, Ph.D., is a clinical psychologist and faculty member in the Department of Epidemiology and Social Medicine, Montefiore Medical Center/Albert Einstein College of Medicine, Bronx, NY. He is the psychosocial coordinator for an integrated primary care and substance abuse treatment program for Montefiore patients and their families and he teaches health psychology graduate students at Albert Einstein. Also, he is on the staff and faculty of the Behavioral Anxiety Disorders Service, Behavioral Medicine Program, Columbia-Presbyterian Medical Center, and practices psychotherapy at the Blanton-Peale Counseling Center, Forest Hills, Queens. He was staff psychologist for the Spellman Center for HIV-Related Disease, St. Clare's Hospital and Health Center, New York.

He received his degree in psychology from Florida State University and interned at New York University Medical Center–Bellevue Hospital, New York. He has also has a master's degree in journalism from Columbia University.

Pergamon General Psychology Series

Editors: **Arnold P. Goldstein,** Syracuse University
Leonard Krasner, Stanford University &
SUNY at Stony Brook

*Out of print in original format. Available in custom reprint edition.